A Cruel Wind

Pandemic Flu in America, 1918-1920

D0841623

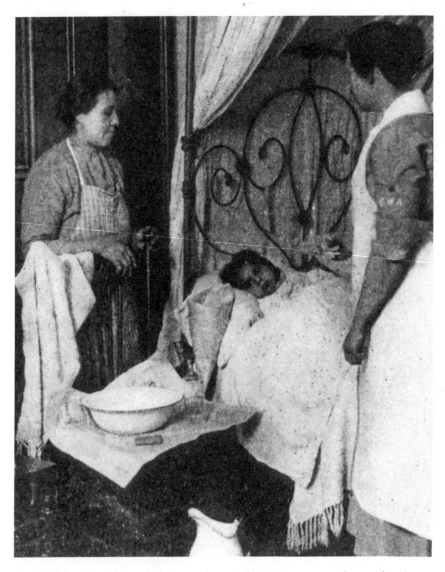

1. A child with influenza, her mother, and a visiting nurse from a local Child Welfare Association

DAVENPORT UNIVERSITY
MIDLAND CAMPUS LIBRARY
3555 EAST PATRICK ROAD
MIDLAND, MI 48642-5837

A Cruel Wind

Pandemic Flu in America, 1918-1920

Dorothy A. Pettit, Ph.D.

and

Janice Bailie, Ph.D.

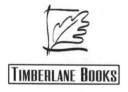

TIMBERLANE BOOKS

MURFREESBORO, TENNESSEE
2008

Copyright © 2008
Timberlane Books
518 Upland Court
Murfreesboro, TN 37129 USA
http://www.timberlanebooks.com

All rights reserved. No part of this book may be reprinted or
reproduced in any form by any electronic, mechanical or other means,
including photocopying and recording in any information storage
or retrieval system, including illustrations, beyond that copying
permitted by Sections 107 and 108 of the U.S. Copyright Law
and except by reviewers for the public press, without
written permission from the copyright holder.

Edited by: R. Neil Scott
                        Middle Tennessee State University

                        Marie F. Harper
                        Los Alamos National Laboratory

Layout & Design by: Sue Balcer
                        www.JustYourType.biz
                        San Antonio, Texas

Indexed by: Sara Lynn Eastler
                        www.AtlanticAuthoring.com
                        Aurora, Colorado

Printed in the United States of America

A catalog record for this book is available from the
Library of Congress.
Library of Congress Control Number: 2008922678

ISBN 978-0-9715428-1-5 [H.C]
ISBN 978-0-9715428-2-2 [Pap.]

To Professor William Greenleaf
D.A.P.

To my aunt, Mrs. Jean Stevenson, for the immeasurable
support she has always given me.
J.B.

Contents

Illustrations

Figures

Tables

Acknowledgements

The authors sincerely appreciate the assistance and many courtesies extended to them by the many archivists and librarians consulted in the process of doing the research for this study, in particular those at: the Yale Sterling Library and Yale Library of Medicine; the Dartmouth Medical Library; the Countway Medical Library; the Rockefeller University Archives; Columbia University's Oral History Division; the Library of the American Philosophical Society in Philadelphia; the National Archives in Washington, D.C. and College Park, Maryland; the Prints and Photographs and Archives Divisions of the Library of Congress; the Johns Hopkins Medical Archives; New York Public Library; the Armed Forces Institute of Pathology; the Wason Collection of the Cornell University Library; and, the National Library of Medicine in Bethesda, Maryland.

Special thanks are extended to Dr. John R. Blake, former Chief of the History of Medicine Division of the National Library of Medicine, for making available the valuable letters written by his father, Dr. Francis G. Blake, during the pandemic period. Dr. Blake's letters are a treasure trove that would help make any history of the pandemic come alive.

We are also indebted to Mrs. Lillian Kidwell, and Rudolph Clemen, formerly with the Archives of the American National Red Cross, Washington, D.C., and the Jenkins family, formerly at the Parsonage Gallery, Durham, New Hampshire. Also, to Carol Fredriksen, formerly with Project HOPE, for her months of hospitality in Washington, D.C.

In addition, we would like to express our gratitude to the various medical specialists and staff at the Centers for Disease Control and Prevention in Atlanta, Georgia, who unselfishly provided time and expertise regarding certain parts of this study.

Another person who was very helpful was Dr. Ira Vaughan Hiscock, M.D., Professor of Public Health, Emeritus, at Yale

University, who read chapters of the dissertation upon which this book is based and offered his wise counsel and encouragement. Also, to Dr. L. Carrington Goodrich, former Professor of History at Columbia University, regarding the impact of the pandemic in China. And, to Dr. Bailie's husband, Mr. Keith Wilson, and her colleague at Sciencewrite, Dr. Heather Anderson, as well as R. Neil Scott of Middle Tennessee State University, and Ms. Marie F. Harper of the Los Alamos National Laboratory, for editing the manuscript.

For supplying photographs, tables and illustrations we thank: Natalie D. Tomasco of the Falvey Memorial Library of Villanova University; Jeffery K. Taubenberger of the Armed Forces Institute of Pathology; Vernon Knight of the Baylor University College of Medicine; Edwin D. Killbourne of New York Medical College; and, David Butler, descendent of Captain Sylvester Benjamin Butler.

All of the above-mentioned research would have been impossible had not the University of New Hampshire provided fellowship and travel funding for the original dissertation and we thank the University for its generous support. We want to also thank the "unsung heroes" at the Reference Desk and in the Inter-Library Loan and Microfilm sections of the Library of the University of New Hampshire for their continued interest and assistance.

Finally, we wish to acknowledge the help of Professor Charles A. Jellison, and the late Professor William Greenleaf, of the Department of History, University of New Hampshire, who served as doctoral advisors and were both encouraging and supportive of the research conducted for the dissertation version of this book.

Dorothy A. Pettit, Ph.D.
Hamden, Connecticut

Janice Bailie, Ph.D.
Belfast, Northern Ireland

A Cruel Wind:
Pandemic Flu in America, 1918-1920

1

The Riddle of Influenza

*Of all the depressing, rotten maladies this takes the cake
and I wonder that anyone has been able to stand being
under the same roof with me for a week. One's many
bad qualities surge to the surface and among the cardinal
symptoms of the disease may be mentioned paralysis
of the hind legs, quarrelsomeness, irritability, loss of
memory, despondency, dislocation of the attachments
of the diaphragm, wasting of the gastrocnemii, and a
hopelessness of spirit. Don't get it.*

So wrote the distinguished neurosurgeon, Harvey Cushing, to
describe his siege of influenza or "grippe" in December 1906.[1]
The acutely perceptive doctor recovered from his affliction that
winter, apparently without complications. A dozen years later, in the
summer of 1918, while serving with the Base Hospitals in France as
Senior Consultant in Neurosurgery of the American Expeditionary
Force, he caught the mysterious malady known as "Spanish flu" or
"three-day grippe." This time, unfortunately, serious complications
did result. Three weeks after his initial attack, Dr. Cushing was still
tottering about and complaining of double vision. An additional
month passed without improvement in his gait—his "hind legs"
noticeably more unsteady each day. Finally came the elevated

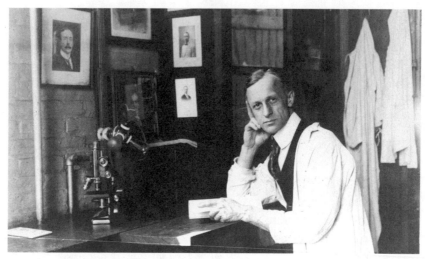

2. Harvey Cushing at his desk at Johns Hopkins.

temperature and loss of sensation in his extremities necessitating a lengthy sojourn in the hospital. The illness, which was eventually diagnosed as vascular polyneuritis, left him a semi-invalid for the rest of his life. Both femoral arteries became permanently occluded, and after 1920 he was unable to walk more than a block or two without stopping to rest. Although a coronary occlusion was the immediate cause of his death in 1939, the most remarkable finding at autopsy was the complete occlusion of his femoral arteries. Considering the "paralysis of the hind legs" and "wasting of the gastrocnemii" (muscles of the lower leg) he complained of in 1906, his vascular damage may have even begun prior to 1918.[2]

Fortunately, not all of the victims of the so-called Spanish flu in 1918 suffered such serious long-term complications as Dr. Cushing. In the spring of that year, an influenza infection was sometimes called a "three-day fever" because of its short duration; however the course of influenza is actually unpredictable.

In most years, influenza is not regarded as a serious illness, but a disease which results in a seasonal increase in respiratory illnesses, with an unfortunate—but expected—increase in mortality among the most vulnerable, usually the very young and the elderly. This book highlights the most frightening characteristic of the virus: its occasional ability to infect huge proportions of the human race. In 1918, Harvey Cushing was lucky enough to recover. In terms of mortality, the influenza pandemic overshadowed World War I.

Diagnosis of influenza may be difficult in the absence of an epidemic, because the clinical signs often lack definitiveness. Usually influenza is characterized by its sudden onset, often in company with chills, severe headache, fever, coryza (acute rhinitis), and cough. Sometimes there is sore throat, muscular pain—especially in the legs and back—sweating, or nausea. Symptoms apparently vary from patient to patient. For instance, military records for the 1918 pandemic showed a sore throat to be an almost universal complaint. But many physicians at the time thought the throats of their patients were rarely involved.[3] Under epidemic conditions, the disease is further characterized by its rapid, even explosive, spread from one individual to another.[4] As for recovery from influenza, with luck patients usually recover in about a week. There may, however, be a residual weakness and depression quite out of proportion to the severity of the disease, especially among adults. Children usually seem to regain their strength more rapidly than their elders.

Why is influenza such a problem? Besides being a difficult disease to diagnose with certainty at the bedside, its prognosis is unpredictable. While the more fortunate victims recover in about a week, rapid death does sometimes occur, usually as a result of pneumonia. Although most view influenza and pneumonia as two separate diseases, occasionally they are not. The term pneumonia, in fact, merely indicates an inflammation in the lungs; it is a disease process rather than a disease. There are more than fifty different causes of pneumonia, the most common being bacteria, viruses, chemical irritants, vegetable dusts, and allergies. Influenza viruses can invade the lungs; if they do, the victim will then have a viral pneumonia. In that case the prognosis must be guarded because antibiotics are often ineffective.

At other times, an influenza victim's recovery may be complicated by the onset of a bacterial pneumonia. In fact, it is theoretically possible for a person to have a viral pneumonia and a bacterial pneumonia at the same time. Indeed, strong and consistent evidence has accumulated indicating clinically important interactions between influenza and bacteria that infect the respiratory tract, including during the 1918 pandemic.[5] One of the bacterial infections most commonly associated with influenza is *Staphylococcus aureus*. Substances called enzymes that are produced by this bacteria are known to cut or cleave one of the influenza virus proteins into two pieces, a necessary step to potentiate infection.[6] In addition, the damage to lung tissue caused by the influenza virus renders the lung more vulnerable to bacterial infection.[7] When simultaneous infection by both viral and bacterial agents is present, antibiotics typically help to clear up the bacterial problem, but that depends on the extent of the infection and the susceptibility of the infecting organism to treatment with antibiotics. Nevertheless, influenza is potentially a grave disease.

In the rest of this chapter, some of the aspects of the influenza riddle will be mentioned briefly. Following a description of viral invasion, replication, and the antigenic structure and component proteins of the virus, there will be discussion of the body's defense system; the developing nomenclature for influenza viruses; the disease in history; the unusual aspects of the 1918 pandemic; and the non-human types of influenza viruses.

First of all, uncomplicated influenza is usually limited to viral involvement of the cells of the upper respiratory tract, the mucous membranes of the nasopharynx (nose and throat), the conjunctiva, and, less often, the lower intestine.[8] If influenza viruses do enter the respiratory system, they usually try to invade the superficial susceptible cells, and it is within those cells that the viruses reproduce, a process taking about six hours. To reproduce, the virus binds to and then enters a living cell, where it commandeers cellular machinery, inducing it to manufacture new copies of the viral components. The pieces then assemble themselves into new viruses that escape the host cell, proceeding to infect other cells. Early research suggested that newly-synthesized viruses leaving the superficial respiratory cells traveled to distant areas of the body, where they, in turn, invaded other body cells, causing the common clinical symptoms reflecting involvement of the central nervous system—a headache, for instance.[9] However, recent research has shown that infection by influenza A in humans is largely confined to the respiratory tract with occasional involvement of the intestinal tract or more occasionally the brain. The clinical symptoms are generally explained by the effect of the immune response to viral infection.[10]

The usual response of the body to infection with a virus is to activate the immune system, which is a cascade of signaling events that ultimately results in the production of protein substances called antibodies. The function of antibodies is to bind to, and neutralize, the invading virus. Should the body experience a further encounter with the same or a similar virus, neutralizing antibodies will again be produced, thus preventing a second attack of the disease. The same antibody response is also provoked by administering a protective vaccine, with the aim of mimicking the action of the natural immune system, giving protection from infection thereafter.

On occasion, as a result of the immune response, influenza viruses are unable to enter the superficial nasopharyngeal cells. Even if some flu viruses do enter the superficial cells, the process of viral replication may not occur. Without viral reproduction, a generalized infection fails to occur. Such a brief encounter with an influenza virus is usually enough to trigger the body's defense mechanism to react against a foreign protein substance, which is what a virus is. Foreign protein substances are called antigens; therefore an invading virus may be considered an antigenic agent which stimulates the host to produce defensive antibodies.

It is important to understand that some viruses are complex antigenic substances. They contain not one, but several, antigenic substances. These antigenic substances vary in importance in determining whether or not the victim will have a clinical case of influenza.

To appreciate the complex antigenic character of the influenza virus, a description of the virus itself is useful. The usually spherical virus particle, which is sometimes referred to as a type of "virion"—a complete virus particle that is structurally intact and infectious[11]—is: seventy-five percent protein, one percent ribonucleic acid (RNA), six-and-a-half percent carbohydrate and approximately eighteen percent lipid. Within the core, or nucleocapsid, of the virion is the ribonucleic acid (RNA), the genetic material of the virus. Related to the viral RNA is the major nucleoprotein (NP) antigen, the antigen used for classifying influenza viruses into Types A, B, and C.[12]

Surrounding the nucleocapsid of the virus are double layers, an inner protein and an outer lipid membrane. On the outer membrane are two types of spike-like projections, glycoproteins called hemagglutinin (H or HA) and neuraminidase (N or NA). These glycoproteins, which are morphologically and antigenically distinct substances, are also major antigens. Their discovery made the classification of influenza viruses into Types A, B, and C inadequate, and they are now used as signature proteins to identify different strains of the virus.[13] There are at least fifteen known variants of the HA protein and nine of the NA protein.[14] Since the identification of the HA and NA antigens, it has become evident that there are still other important protein substances within viruses.[15] A description of these will be useful in understanding how the virus enters the human system and exploits the body's own cells to perpetuate itself.

In fact, the influenza virus comprises eight genes, each of which gives rise to one or more proteins – at least ten are known. The protein products of each gene have a role to play in the influenza virus' functions and activities.

For infection by influenza virus to occur, the HA protein must bind to receptors called sialic acids on the host cell surface.

The specific receptors differ between species, which determines the type of host the virus is able to infect. For the HA protein to be activated within the host cell, it must be cut or cleaved into two pieces, and the virus generally uses the host's own cellular proteins, called enzymes, to achieve this. Enzymes are proteins which exert their activity on other proteins or molecules such as DNA or RNA, bringing about a change: for example, in the shape of a molecule, breaking up a molecule; or possibly, manufacturing new copies of a molecule.

Any changes in the HA protein sequence may allow the virus to recognize and infect a new host or even a different species, as even a small change in the protein sequence can lead to a radical change in the shape of the molecule. The influenza virus is characterized by the frequency with which those changes occur, and they can be minor (usually referred to as antigenic *drift*) or quite major (usually referred to as antigenic *shift*). Antigenic shift in one or more of the viral surface antigens is known to be a trigger for an influenza viral strain to infect a new species or many individuals on a pandemic scale.

The neuraminidase (NA) protein enables new virus copies to escape the host cell so they can subsequently infect other cells. Also an enzyme, the NA protein has the ability to cleave the target sialic acid receptors from viruses newly emerging or budding from the surface of infected cells, releasing the virus particles to proceed with the invasion of further cells. The neuraminidase protein has become an important target for antiviral drugs. If the release of viruses for further infection can be prevented by use of neuraminidase inhibitors (such as oseltamivir – Tamiflu™), this can prevent the spread of the virus throughout the cells of the respiratory system.

The NS1 gene encodes two proteins, NS1 and NS2 (NEP). The non-structural (NS1) protein is known to have important effects on the immune system of the host, suppressing the interferon α/β system, which is an early warning system activated during the initial response of the host to viral infection. This system is described in more detail below. Having the ability to suppress or block the response gives the virus time immediately after infection to establish itself and replicate without interference from the immune response of the host. Experimental results suggest that the NS1 protein from the 1918 pandemic virus was especially efficient at blocking the interferon response. Less is known about the function of the NS2 protein.

Also making up a major portion of the viral protein are membrane proteins M1 and M2, which have a number of important functions relating to the movement and reproduction of the virus.

The nucleoprotein (NP) gene is known to be involved in many aspects of viral function and is highly conserved. This protein, which is the major structural component of the nucleocapsid, is known to interact with host proteins, and as such, like HA and NA, is another important determinant of host specificity.

The remaining three genes of the influenza virus are called polymerase genes: PA, PB1 and PB2. Enzymes encoded by those genes are very important because they act upon the viral genes, making copies of the virus' genetic material. Some types of polymerase (e.g. human DNA polymerase), have proofreading activity, which actually corrects any errors that occur while DNA is being copied or replicated, and thus prevents genetic changes from occurring. Such activity is vital for survival of a complex organism such as a mammal. However, the influenza RNA polymerases lack such proofreading activity, which explains the ease with which the influenza virus acquires genetic changes. As discussed, that is an advantage for the virus, enabling it to evade the immune system of a host that possesses antibodies against a previous version of the virus. Importantly, it has been noted that the three polymerase genes are often cotransmitted with the HA gene, and in the case of the 1918 pandemic strain, were likely to have contributed to the rapidity with which the virus was able to reproduce itself once inside the body.[16]

Influenza viruses, then, are complex antigenic agents, which stimulate the host to produce defensive antibodies. But antibodies are not the only substance produced by the body in response to the invasion of flu viruses. The process set in motion when influenza viruses enter the nasopharyngeal cavity is a highly complicated phenomenon that is still not completely understood. Influenza viruses are unlike bacteria in that the cells of the victim, or host, are indispensable in the virus' reproductive process. Bacteria, such as streptococci may enter the cells of victims, but they do not require the aid of host cells to duplicate. The influenza virus must enter the host cell to reproduce. What happens within the host cell is shown in figure 1.1.[17]

Figure 1.1 Time sequence of influenza virus replication:

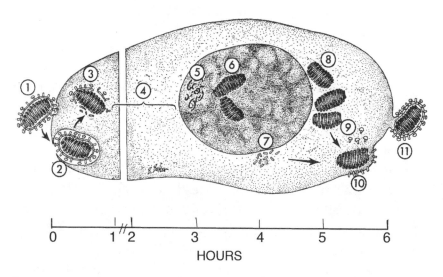

Time sequence of influenza virus replication: (1) adsorption, (2) penetration, (3) uncoating, (4) eclipse, (5) viral nucleoprotein antigen pieces (intranuclear), (6) viral nucleoprotein helix, (7) hemagglutinin, (8) cytoplasmic ribonucleoprotein, (9) neuraminidase is formed in the cytoplasm, (10) budding virus, and (11) pedunculated virus, viral outer coat continuous with host cell membrane.

As figure 1.1 demonstrates, the virus breaks up into protein fragments after entering a respiratory cell, and then is reassembled. Multiplication of the virus, perhaps as much as a one-hundred-fold increase in approximately five hours, also takes place within the cell. Then the newly-synthesized viral particles go forth to infect other cells, causing cell destruction in the process.[18]

Thus influenza viruses lack independence because of their special relationship with the cells of the host. Those host cells have a vital role to play in the infective process and in the life cycle of the virus. If an influenza virus is going to cause a case of flu, for instance, it must first find a host cell with suitable receptors on its surface. Next, the virus must penetrate the cell membrane, a process that often involves a compatibility of the lipoproteins of both virus and cell. Then, once inside, the viral RNA is synthesized within the nucleus of the cell.[19] Finally, the reassembled virus particle acquires a lipid envelope or membrane, during the budding stage, of host-cell origin (see figure 1.1). Consequently, viral infection depends upon cooperative host cells.

In addition, host cells produce a protein substance, unrelated to antibody production, in response to viral invasion. This substance, called interferon, is produced almost immediately in response to viral infection, and plays a critical role in arresting the reproduction of viruses within the cells. However, interferon does not protect cells from infection by viruses. Instead, it is rapidly released by the infected cell and binds to specific receptors on surrounding cells, upregulating many genes (>100) that constitute an antiviral response.[20] In this manner, the interferon early warning system aids in preventing synthesis of new viral particles. As previously discussed, the influenza NS1 protein (and possibly other proteins such as the viral polymerases), antagonize the interferon response. The viral NS1 protein is known to bind to and sequester double-stranded RNA produced during viral replication, thus perhaps concealing the presence of the virus from the host.[21] Recently, scientists have discovered other mechanisms by which the influenza virus can evade the host immune response, by interacting with proteins within the host cell that may lead to death of the invading immune cells.[22] The interferon response mechanism seems to promote a biological paradox: studies indicate that the double-stranded RNA (dsRNA) produced during replication of the virus—which stimulates the production of interferon—may actually hasten the destruction or death of uninfected cells and increase the toxic effects of the viral infection.[23] However, the sacrifice of those cells might be seen as an attempt by the body to starve the virus of vessels in which to replicate. In the early stages of infection by influenza, then, the virus plays a cat-and-mouse game with the immune system of the host.

The 1918 virus was able to replicate at an astonishing speed and rapidly overwhelm an immune system. In response to that, the victim's body mounted an uncontrolled exuberant immune response, in a desperate attempt to halt the progress of the virus in the lungs, typically accompanied by a characteristic blue-black coloring of the face, particularly in the lips, ears, and extremities (heliotrope cyanosis), as victims struggled for breath while their lungs filled up with fluid, blood and inflammatory cells. This phenomenon—the exaggerated immune response—is now described as a cytokine storm, and the resulting suffocation is recognized by modern medicine as acute respiratory distress syndrome (ARDS).[24]

Many aspects of the behavior of the influenza virus puzzled scientists following the 1918 pandemic, and while answers to some of these questions have been found, the virus still presents many challenges for modern-day epidemiologists and molecular geneticists.

A further complication in the story of the body's defense mechanism against the influenza virus for researchers of 1918 was the puzzling way the antibody system operated. Many viruses, including the measles virus, stimulate the production of enough lasting antibodies to prevent reinfection. One infection with the measles virus, whether natural or vaccine-induced, usually prevents future attacks. The antibody production provoked by the influenza virus, however, seems to have only limited effectiveness, probably because so many variant strains were circulating. Moreover, the antibodies first produced in response to influenza may be those most effective against a prior flu infection, a phenomenon sometimes referred to as the "doctrine of original antigenic sin."[25] It would appear that one's strongest antibody response relates to the strain of influenza first encountered in one's youth, rather than to the current invading strain.

In 1968, for example, young children who were infected by the new "Hong Kong" influenza virus produced large numbers of antibodies against it, but children between ten and twelve, when attacked by the same "Hong Kong" strain, produced greater quantities of antibodies against the 1957 "Asian flu" virus. The ten to twelve year-olds eventually produced effective antibodies against the 1968 virus as well, but their highest antibody response was to the virus prevalent in their childhood.[26] This phenomenon repeated itself in every other age group—the very elderly are thought to have been protected from the 1968 pandemic by virtue of their experience with the same subtype of HA antigens as children.[27] This seems to be an inefficient defense system and may explain the occurrence of successive pandemic outbreaks of the virus. Some scientists suggested that the body's antibody response to influenza may be the result of an "immunologic memory," or that perhaps it is genetically programmed. Such concepts are now well recognized and documented as our understanding of the immune system has developed.[28]

Equally puzzling for scientists of 1918 was the fact that the virus apparently did not always make exact copies of itself. Laboratory studies showed that the virus particles emerging from the host cell after synthesis could have a different structural makeup from that of the invading virus. It seemed clear to scientists studying influenza that the process by which new viral strains emerged was partially controlled by man himself. His cells certainly played an active role in the proliferation of viruses, and those same cells may have helped to determine the antigenic nature of the strains in circulation. One scientist has even speculated that the influenza virus might be a tool of the body used to send messages from cell to cell and that variations of the virus represent the evolution of the host cell rather than the virus.[29]

We know now that the emergence of these new strains may occur in a variety of ways. During replication of the viral RNAs by the three error-prone polymerase enzymes, genetic changes known as mutations can occur. Some of these may have little or no effect on the resultant viral protein produced, or the change may be a particularly important one that allows the virus to acquire a new characteristic. More major changes can occur if, for example, the host cell is exposed to two different viral strains, when the emergent virus particles may be a combination of the two, rather than exact replications of the invaders. This process of reassortment is now known to be a possible opportunity for the virus to cross the species barrier: for example, when a human infected with influenza is in close proximity to swine which are infected with a different strain. Because the population would lack immunity to the new combination, the new reassembled virus would then have the capacity to cause widespread disease.

Many virologists do not believe, however, that new strains of influenza viruses make their appearance at particular points in time, infect the population and then vanish, never to be encountered again.[30] They believe instead that there are a finite number of possible protein fragment combinations that can occur within a cell, and there has been some evidence that those combinations may even recur in a somewhat cyclic pattern.[31] As yet, there may not have been enough pandemics since the identification of the virus for that question to be answered. Is there, in fact, a pattern to antigenic construction? Or, will time prove them to be merely random selections?

Actually, scientific knowledge about influenza viruses

dates back to only the 1930s. In 1918, most scientists believed that respiratory diseases were the result of infection with one of a number of bacterial agents. A theory that was regarded with much skepticism at the time had been put forward by a pair of French and British research teams, who suggested that the agent was probably a filterable virus.[32]

While research at the time attempted to confirm the causative agent, the first to successfully isolate a human influenza virus was the British research team of Wilson Smith, Christopher H. Andrewes, and Patrick P. Laidlaw.[33] Their 1933 discovery marked the culmination of fifteen years of international scientific endeavor to find the cause of influenza.[34] However, within twenty years of the British findings, it became apparent that there were *many* influenza viruses; "many" in the sense that their structure and antigenic content varied. In 1947, for instance, scientists found a third (NP) antigen. Consequently, what was needed was some orderly system of nomenclature to explain the antigenic variation. The earliest classification system adopted was a product of the World Health Organization (WHO). WHO decided that influenza viruses should be described according to the (NP) antigen. As a result, the new nomenclature was simple: Type A, B, and C viruses. In addition to a description of the (NP) antigen, the name of the virus was to contain the place of origin, the strain serial number, and the year of isolation. An example of the recommended nomenclature was the name given to the 1957 "Asian flu" strain: A/Singapore/1/57.[35]

This simple nomenclature was adequate through the 1950s, when virologists believed that the envelope surrounding the core of the virus contained a single antigenic substance, the hemagglutinin (HA) antigen. However, when virologists discovered the existence of the neuraminidase (NA) antigen in the 1960s, the classification of influenza viruses into Types A, B, and C no longer seemed adequate. Strains of Type A viruses apparently could contain new HA or NA antigens on their surfaces, and sometimes both changed at once.

For example, between 1933 and 1957 the strains now

identified as H1N1 were in circulation, although those strains circulating before 1947, when a significant antigenic drift occurred, were previously termed H0N1. Since nomenclature was updated in 1980, H0 is no longer regarded as a distinct subtype. In 1957, however, a viral strain emerged with changes in both outer antigens. Thus, the modern name for the 1957 pandemic strain is now: A/Singapore/1/57 (H2N2). The NA antigen that appeared in 1957 is still circulating, but the HA antigen changed again in 1968, and the current pool of circulating strains still contains H3N2 strains. Most recently, scientists have become concerned that a strain of avian influenza (H5N1) has the potential to cross the species barrier and possibly cause a new pandemic among humans.

Why is it important to know about antigenic changes in the virus? Because when major antigenic changes occur, widespread epidemics of influenza result. Indeed, such epidemics are called pandemics because they are worldwide. Because large numbers of people everywhere have no antibodies in their systems against the new antigen, the virus finds it easy to enter a victim's respiratory system and begin to replicate.

In the mid-1970s it was noted that pandemic influenza *seemed* to occur about every ten years or so. That belief had become so firmly established in the influenza literature, that in February 1976, the *New York Times* published an editorial highlighting the fact that influenza pandemics had, "…marked the end of every decade – every eleven years, since the 1940s."[36] The theory resulted in a number of scares, such as the cases in Fort Dix in 1976 that led to an unnecessary national immunization campaign, and the rumors about the Russian flu epidemic that threatened to go global in 1977.[37] Fortunately, no major true influenza A pandemic has occurred since 1968, and given the intervals between those that *have* happened, it can be stated that no predictable pattern of pandemic periodicity exists.[38]

Influenza is still a problem between pandemics. Between the major *shifts* in the antigenic nature of the virus in circulation, new viral strains emerge representing *drifts* in the antigenic material.

The drifts exhibit minor structural changes, but do not alter the HA and NA antigens attached to the outer layer of the virus. Drifts in the antigenic makeup of the virus usually cause epidemics or local outbreaks rather than pandemics, although they, too, can be somewhat global in distribution.[39]

It is the group of Type A viruses that apparently causes pandemic influenza. The term *pandemic* now refers to influenza outbreaks exhibiting changes in the HA and/or NA antigens. Inter-pandemic outbreaks of influenza may be recurring epidemics of the pandemic strain, or drifts from the pandemic strain.

In his essay, "A Virologist's Perspective," Edwin D. Kilbourne identified seven pandemics, pseudopandemics and pandemic threats that have occurred since 1933.[40] Table 1.1 lists the incidents he identified.

The Type B viruses seem to have less antigenic variation than the As, but Bs also cause epidemic influenza. Epidemics caused by B strains seem to occur less frequently, however, than those caused by A strains. The Type C virus (which has been isolated) usually does not cause detectable disease in man, although much of the population demonstrates through the presence of antibodies a previous acquaintance with it.

Shortly after the postulation of the "doctrine of original antigenic sin" in 1953—the theory that antibody production, particularly against the HA antigen, was greatest against the strain or subtype of influenza circulating in one's early years—scientists found evidence to suggest that antigenic variation might occur in a cyclic pattern. In 1957 some laboratory studies on the era of people who were young children around 1890, reported the presence of antibodies against the (H2) antigen of the 1957 "Asian flu" virus. Although several other studies did not back that finding absolutely, it sparked the theory that the (H2) antigen had circulated in the past. Stronger support for the cyclic theory came again in 1968, when it was found that elderly people born in

Table 1.1 Pandemics, pseudo-pandemics and pandemic threats, 1947-1999[41]

1947 – Influenza 'A Prime' – a global, relatively non-lethal epidemic of a variant virus of the same A subtype that had circulated since 1929. Vaccines made from antecedent (H1N1) strains failed to protect.

1957 – The first true pandemic since 1918. The H2N2 Asian influenza virus differed from its antecedents in both major antigens, thus confronting the world's population with an essentially novel virus to which it had no immunity. This epidemic was important in demonstrating that a 'modern' influenza virus could cause pandemic disease and fatal viral pneumonia reminiscent of 1918. Completely replaced all H1N1 subtype viruses.

1968 – In the 'Hong Kong' pandemic only the major haemagglutinin (HA) antigen changed, but change was sufficient to induce a pandemic, modified in severity by population immunity against the minor neuraminidase (NA) antigen. Completely replaced all H2N2 viruses.

1976 – At least 250 recruits at Fort Dix, New Jersey were infected with swine influenza virus. A controversial mass immunization program was initiated in the USA for fear of 'another 1918'. With no further cases of disease and complications attributed to the vaccine, the program was cancelled after vaccination of 43 million people.

1977 – The Russian flu (actually originating in China) which produced a global pandemic affecting initially those less that 25 years of age. An early return of a virus (H1N1) last seen two decades before. Unprecedented co-circulation of H1N1 and H3N2 (Hong Kong) subtypes continue to this day.

1997 – H5N1 avian influenza in Hong Kong with sixteen-proved infections of humans and six fatalities. Perhaps due to mass destruction of chickens suspected to be the source, the epidemic ceased.

1999 – H9N2 avian virus appeared early in the year, also in Hong Kong, as a brief zoonotic infection without evidence of human to human transmission. As with H5N1 virus, apparent origin in chickens. Apparent cessation of cases without mass slaughter of fowl.

the late 1800s had antibodies reacting with the 1968 (H3) "Hong Kong" strain. It was reported that those born between 1898 and 1900 had those antibodies circulating in their bodies even before the new 1968 (H3N2) virus appeared.[42] Most recent laboratory results and epidemiological evidence tends to confirm that there is strong evidence for recycling of the H3 antigen (which has now been strongly linked to the 1890 pandemic), but the evidence for recycling of H2 antigens is not clear, and there is no compelling evidence for recycling of H1 antigens.[43]

While the cyclic behavior of circulating influenza virus strains may still be a puzzle, there is no question that the disease known as influenza is an old affliction, as in the historical sense. Influenza has long fascinated students interested in the history and geography of disease, particularly because serious respiratory epidemics—in terms of fatalities—have been a recurrent phenomenon. A major problem for medical historians, however, has been the interpretation of old records. Symptoms and the clinical course of many of the recorded diseases are often so vague and incomplete that it is impossible to distinguish between influenza, for instance, and pneumonic plague.

The written history of influenza probably starts in the Middle Ages. Influenza pandemics (meaning many deaths occurred) have been found to have occurred during 1173 in the areas comprising modern-day Italy, Germany, and England. The same countries had two serious respiratory epidemics in the fourteenth century and three in the next century. Historians also suggest that the astrological designation "influenza," or "influence of the stars," dates back to the fourteenth century, although the name was uncommon until the eighteenth century.[44]

During the fifteenth and sixteenth centuries, Italian physicians recorded five serious epidemics of pulmonary disease.

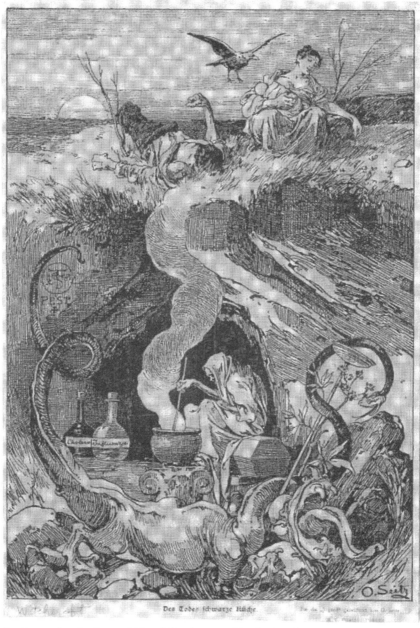

3. Poster by O. Seitz, 1896: "Cholera and Influenza"

Because the death toll each time was high, Italian diagnosticians described the disease as pneumonic plague. Recent scholars have discounted the diagnosis of plague in those early epidemics, however, for the mortality rates seem to have been in the range of about ten to thirty percent. Had pneumonic plague been the disease in circulation, the fatality rates would have been eighty percent or better. (Before the advent of antibiotics, pneumonic plague was a highly fatal disease.) Nineteenth and twentieth century medical historians have decided that the Italian episodes were probably outbreaks of influenzal pneumonia.[45]

It is possible, of course, that medieval physicians used the word "plague" to describe any epidemic with a high mortality. In that sense influenza sometimes *is* a "pneumonic plague." While it is recognized that—during pandemic episodes—many people die from the pneumonic process in their lungs, the use of the category of "pneumonic plague" today refers to a specific disease caused by bacteria, not viruses. The disease now known as plague, in either bubonic or pneumonic form, was found to be the result of infection by an organism called *Pasteurella pestis* (now known as *Yersinia pestis*).[46] Since the discovery of the *Pasteurella* organism in 1894, the diagnosis of plague has been specific. But the use of the word "plague" to describe any serious disease was still common for many years after that, especially during the 1918 influenza pandemic.

An example of the problem medical historians have had in trying to trace episodes of influenza is shown in the vagueness of information detailed in *Virus and Rickettsial Diseases with Especial Consideration of Their Public Health Significance* (see Table 1.2). When Dr. John Mote put the table together in 1940, he used the term *pandemic* to describe only the episodes of influenza having high fatality rates and those that seemed to travel rapidly through the inhabited parts of the world.[47]

Table 1.2 Historic epidemics and pandemics of influenza

1510	First well-described European influenza epidemic
1557	Epidemic coming from Far East and spreading over Europe
1580	*First pandemic* beginning in the Far East and spreading over Europe (no record in America)
1593	Epidemic limited to Europe
1647	*First American epidemic*, limited to Western Hemisphere
1655-1658	Epidemic starting in America in 1655 and spreading to Europe
1675	Epidemic in England and France (? of influenza)
1698	Epidemic limited to North America
1709-1712	Severe epidemic period limited to Eastern Hemisphere
1729-1733	*World pandemic* occurring in successive waves and spreading from east to west
1757-1762	Epidemic starting in North America and spreading to South America and Europe
1767	Epidemic concurrent in North America and Europe
1772	Epidemic limited to Western Hemisphere
1775-1776	Epidemic limited to England and parts of Europe
1780-1782	Epidemic in North America, 1780, spreading to Europe, and finally becoming *pandemic* in Russia in 1782
1788-1790	*Severe pandemic* starting in Prussia and spreading west
1798-1803	Severe epidemic starting in North America and spreading east
1830-1833	*Pandemic* starting in China and spreading west
1836-1837	*Pandemic* starting in Russia and spreading south and west
1847-1850	*Pandemic* of undetermined origin
1857-1858	Epidemic on both hemispheres
1873-1875	Epidemic limited to Western Hemisphere
1889	World *pandemic* starting in the Far East and spreading west
1918	World *pandemic* of questionable origin

But Mote's chart omitted many other epidemics of influenza recorded in history. For instance, Thomson and Thomson's two-volume monograph on influenza, which was published in the 1930s, mentioned epidemics in America in 1811, 1815-16, and 1824-26.[48] Today, historians of influenza would probably be more inclined to include those nineteenth century epidemics in their compilations, for they would want to investigate how often pandemics occur and if they occur in cycles.

Mote also tried to trace the chronology of epidemics and pandemics. Generally the early pandemics were recorded as starting in the Far East, moving west into Russia or traveling via the great trade routes to the bustling ports of eastern and western Europe, and thence to the Western Hemisphere. Influenza was a disease that traveled east to west, probably originating in some obscure Chinese village. The great pandemic of 1889-90 was suggested as having started in Bokhara, Turkistan, or in China; perhaps simultaneously in both places.[49] On the other hand, Greenland had an early epidemic in 1889. But in 1918 many medical authorities still believed China to be the real home of influenza. When China evidently suffered less severely from influenza in the fall of 1918, the Western editor of the *China Medical Journal* thought the Chinese were so familiar with influenza that they possessed an immunity other peoples lacked. China, he thought, was, in fact, the "fountain head of epidemic diseases."[50]

Since the Mote and Thomson and Thomson studies, American medical historians have delved into the history of epidemic diseases in the colonial period of the country, using more traditional historical sources—letters, diaries, etc. Those sources seem to suggest that pandemics of respiratory diseases did indeed occur regularly in ten-to-fifteen-year cycles. Although those documents present certain problems to the historian—the difficulty of trying to distinguish between "pleuretical disorders," "peripneumonias," and influenza, for example—they nonetheless indicate that serious epidemics of respiratory disease occurred regularly throughout the early history of the country.[51]

22

According to American medical historian John Duffy, the first influenza epidemic in North America probably occurred in 1647, when John Winthrop recorded the following observations:

> An epidemical sickness was through the country among the Indians and English, French and Dutch. It took them like a cold, and light fever with it. Such as bled or used cooling drinks died; those who took comfortable things, for the most part recovered, and that in a few days. Wherein a special providence of God appeared, for not a family, nor but few persons escaping it, had it brought all so weak as it brought some, and continued so long, such was the mercy of God to his people, as few died, not above forty or fifty in the Massachusetts, and nearly as many at Connecticut.[52]

Similar epidemics evidently occurred in the 1660s, but the numbers of fatalities were either unremarkable or not recorded. Another "general catarrh" swept Western Europe and North America about 1675.[53] The next pandemic was evidently more severe, striking England and Ireland in 1688 and Virginia the following year. That time the outbreak was so serious that "the people dyed...as in a plague."[54] Curiously, the Virginia epidemic seemed to affect only that colony, or simply went undocumented in the others.

After a period of about ten years, influenza reappeared in the colonies in 1697, and Cotton Mather took pen in hand to record its existence in January of 1699:

> The sickness...extended to allmost all families. Few or none escaped, and many dyed especially in Boston, and some dyed in a strange and unusual manner, in some families all weer sick together so that it was a time of distress.[55]

The 1697-99 viral strain was, apparently, unusually lethal. For example, in Fairfield, Connecticut, seventy people out of a population of fewer than a thousand died within a three month period. Fortunately, few other colonial towns recorded such high mortality rates.[56]

Duffy's colonial research indicates that the next "mortal sickness" of a respiratory character occurred about ten or eleven years later in 1711-12, and that Virginia had yet, another "sickly time" in the early 1720s.[57] Those early historical records show that a "winter disease" (most likely influenza) came about every ten years or so, just as in modern time, when major shifts in the antigenic nature of the influenza virus occurred in 1947, 1957, and 1968.

The Mote chart also suggests that no serious epidemics or pandemics occurred between 1889 and 1918, or for approximately thirty years. Since Mote's time, however, investigators of American epidemics have found a considerable number of influenza epidemics recorded during that thirty-year period. Table 1.3, from Knight, (ed.), *Viral and Mycoplasmal Infections of the Respiratory Tract* (1973), lists a series of epidemics between the pandemics of 1889 and 1918.[58]

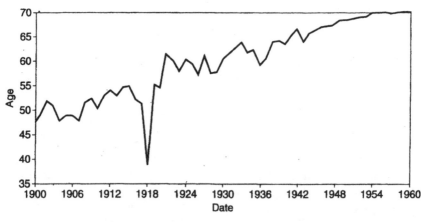

Figure 1.2 Life expectancy in the United States, 1900-60, showing drop in 1918 due to the "Spanish Flu."

Table 1.3: Epidemics and pandemics of influenza United States—1889 to 1969

*Year	Description of Outbreak	Etiology †Influenza A	‡Influenza B
1889-1895	Pandemic	A/Asian-like virus? (H2N?)	
1886, 1897	Epidemics	Etiology unknown	
1889, 1900	Large epidemics	A/Hong Kong (H3?)	
		A/H equi 2 N equi 2 and H2N?	
1901, 1903, 1905, 1907, 1908, 1910, 1915, 1916, 1917,			
1918	Epidemics	Etiology unknown	
1918-1920	Pandemic	A/swine-like virus (Hsw1N1)?	
1922	Epidemic		B?
1923, 1926	Epidemics	A/swine-like virus (Hsw1N1)?	
1928	Epidemic		B?
1929, 1931	Epidemics	A/swine-like virus (Hsw1N1)?	
1932	Epidemic		B?
1933, 1935	Epidemics	A/PR/8-like strains (HON1)	
1936	Epidemic		B?
1937, 1939	Epidemics	A/derivative (HON1)	
1940	Epidemic		B LEE
1941, 1944	Epidemics	A/derivative (HON1)	
1945	Epidemic		B1 BON, KRI
1946, 1947	Epidemics	A/FM1 (H1N1)	
1950, 1951	Epidemics		B1 BON-like
1951, 1953	Epidemics	A/derivative (H1N1)	
1957-1958	Pandemic	A/Asian (H2N2)	
1960	Epidemic	A/Asian derivative (H2N2)	
1962	Epidemic		B2
1963, 1965, 1966	Epidemics	A/Asian derivative (H2N2)	
1966	Epidemic		B2
1968	Epidemic	A/Asian dervative (H2N2)	
1968-1969	Pandemic	A/Hong Kong (H3N2)	
1969	Epidemic		B2

* Outbreaks listed before 1910 are data from Massachusetts (Collins, S. D., and Lehmann J.: Excess deaths from influenza and pneumonia and from important chronic diseases during epidemic periods, 1918-1951. *Public Health Monographs, No. 10*, 1953.)

† Designation of outbreaks of type A influenza before 1933, indicated by question marks are from Masurel, N.: Serological characteristics of a "new" serotype of influenza A virus: the Hong Kong strain. *Bull. WHO*, 41:461, 1969.

‡ Type B outbreaks before 1940, indicated by questions marks, were predicted by the Commission on Acute Respiratory Diseases (*Amer. J. Hygiene*, 43:29, 1946).

A few reasons might be offered to explain Mote's omission of the epidemics that occurred between 1889 and 1918. In the first place, Mote decided to include only those epidemics that seemed to have global significance and which were marked by high fatality rates. The fatality rates of the epidemics in the United States after 1889 were apparently unremarkable. But perhaps a more compelling reason for Mote's omission has to do with the medical community's approach to influenza during the period from 1889 to 1918. Shortly after the pandemic of 1889, the noted European bacteriologist, Richard Friedrich Johannes Pfeiffer, identified a bacillus (a rod-shaped bacterium) as the causative organism in influenza. Pfeiffer's organism, which is sometimes called the Pfeiffer bacillus or the influenza bacillus, is properly designated *Hemophilus influenzae*. Pfeiffer's discovery led some physicians to believe that bacilli were the cause of influenza epidemics.[59]

Pfeiffer, of course, represented the medical scientist in the Age of Bacteriology, which began about 1875. All diseases had natural causes, and bacteria were the primary cause of disease. As such, it was the mission of the scientist to discover those bacteria, and then to find a cure or antidote. Since the Pfeiffer bacillus was blameless in influenza, the disease often went undiagnosed or misdiagnosed after 1892. Certainly when the mysterious "Spanish flu" began to sweep the world in 1918, many physicians believed Pfeiffer's bacillus was its cause.

The etiology of influenza was, indeed, one of the most serious and frustrating problems to arise in 1918. Equally puzzling was the relationship between influenza and pneumonia. Influenza bacilli had been found so often in throat cultures that they had come to be associated only with upper respiratory infections. Influenza bacilli seemed to cause only minor respiratory disease. The disease known as pneumonia, on the other hand, which was often fatal, was the result of infection by another type of bacteria called pneumococci. Pneumococci so often caused serious lung infections that the very name signified they produced disease in the lungs. Actually, however,

Hemophilus influenzae, pneumococci, and many other bacteria can cause pneumonia.

When the pandemic of 1918 began, some medical scientists were also unaware that there was a "normal flora" of bacteria in the mouth. Their view of bacteria was that they were disease producers. Consequently, when so many of the throat cultures made from ailing soldiers and sailors grew out influenza bacilli and different types of pneumococci, the laboratory staff thought those organisms were responsible for the ongoing disease process. It was not until the spring of 1919, for instance, that bacteriologists at the Rockefeller Institute in New York City discovered that perfectly healthy individuals, about thirty percent of a control group, harbored influenza bacilli in their naso-pharyngeal area.[60]

Breath-borne measles was the most common cause of pneumonia epidemics in the Army prior to 1918, and sometimes caused the death of young recruits.[61] One of the first observations made by those who were studying the serious pneumonia problem in the nation's Army camps in early 1918 was that pneumococci did not seem to be causing the pneumonias. Instead of pneumococci, streptococci seemed to be at fault. As a result the pneumococcal vaccine, which had been the only vaccine developed to combat pneumonia, was going to have a limited value. The story of the 1918 influenza pandemic is as much the story of pneumonia as influenza, for almost everyone who died from the pandemic disease had a pneumonia of viral or bacterial origin.[62]

Another mystery in 1918 was where and how the pandemic began. The earliest epidemics of the so-called "Spanish flu" seemed to erupt simultaneously or in rapid succession on three continents— Europe, North America, and Asia. In the United States the first epidemics seemed to break out in March and April at the Army camps and among the Navy personnel along the east coast. But while these outbreaks were in process, highly contagious influenza was claiming many victims in France—and in China. But medical records for China were almost nonexistent (and hardly reliable to the Western expert) in 1918.[63]

Because the earliest epidemics apparently occurred simultaneously in the United States and in France, epidemiologists began to question seriously the theory that China was the seedbed of pandemic influenza. For many years after the 1918 pandemic the theory that pandemic influenza probably had multiple foci of origin became popular. Influenza watchers gradually accepted the idea that the next great pandemic would appear simultaneously all over the world. It would have multiple foci of origin.

But influenza was not a reportable disease in the early months of 1918; physicians did not report cases of influenza to local or state boards of health. Perhaps the earliest cases of influenza only appear to have started among the Army and Navy personnel because the military records were, with few exceptions, the only records kept of outbreaks of influenza. All the military records actually point out is that epidemics of influenza did erupt early in 1918. The records should not be interpreted to mean that pandemic influenza seeded itself in the Army camps and only then infected the civilian sector. The real problem for the student of the pandemic is that so few records of respiratory epidemics were kept in the early months of 1918. Yet the U.S. mortality rates for the spring of 1918 show unmistakably that many urban areas across the nation had high death rates during March and April. Army, Navy and civilian populations probably had concurrent epidemics in early 1918. In the wake of the 1918 pandemic, however, China seemed to be absolved.

Perhaps even more puzzling than where the pandemic originated was its peculiar mortality pattern. During the 1918 pandemic the virus was somewhat selective. About fifty percent of those who died were between twenty and forty years of age. Influenza and pneumonia death rates for 15 to 34 year-olds were more than 20 times higher in 1918 than in previous years; they were people in the prime of life, a group that usually has a very low death rate from influenza.[64] Those studying epidemics and pandemics often consider the excess death rate attributed to influenza (that is, the increase in death rate over the expected average for the time of year). In 1918-1919, those under 65 accounted for more than 99 percent of all excess influenza-related deaths. In contrast, during the 1957 and 1968 pandemics, people under 65 accounted for only 36 percent and 48 percent, respectively, of excess influenza-related deaths.[65] In 1918, people of all ages were attacked by the virus; in fact, the highest incidence was, as usual, in the age group of five to fourteen. However in that group the mortality rate was low. Fatalities were too often soldiers, pregnant women, and healthy young war-workers; children were more apt to lose their parents than their grandparents.[66]

Medical scientists in 1918 had no explanation for such a mortality pattern. Those who had lived through the 1889-90 pandemic recalled that in 1889 most of the fatalities were the older members of society. Why were the young adults so affected this time? There were no answers, only awareness that history was repeating itself. During an emergency meeting of medical experts in the fall of 1918, Dr. Hermann M. Biggs, New York State Commissioner of Health, told those in attendance that the 1918 pandemic resembled the pandemic of 1830-33 in that it took the lives of so many young adults.[67] His remarks seem to suggest that there may also be a cycle in mortality patterns. The curious mortality pattern of the 1918 pandemic remains to be fully explained. One speculative theory is that a somewhat similar strain had been in circulation prior to 1889, and exposure to that strain provided partial protection for those who had encountered it.[68] Unfortunately, in the absence of any pathology specimens taken from human influenza victims during nineteenth century pandemics, the hypothesis cannot be confirmed.

Wartime conditions in 1918 may have affected, to some degree, the unusual mortality pattern. Society was on the move. Scores of young people had left their rural surroundings to move to the large industrial centers for work in defense plants. Young men in the service, particularly those from the country, were exposed to a host of bacterial and viral agents they had never encountered before. The increase in infectious diseases, especially respiratory diseases, was a natural by-product of war.

But World War I was not responsible for another unusual aspect of the 1918 variety of flu—the severe after-effects of the pandemic disease. Although influenza is normally a short-term illness, in 1918 many victims were ill for months. Some people never completely regained their health. Often accompanying the pandemic disease were complications (such as pneumonia) and long-term sequelae (such as loss of smell and taste). In other instances it was reported that victims' hair turned white, or even fell out due to the high fever associated with the disease.[69] During the 1918 pandemic many victims had vascular damage; still others had impaired central nervous systems. Some of the damage was minor. People complained of excessive fatigue or perhaps a lack of appetite. But other victims had neuralgias, polyneuritis, and even psychoses. Still others had tachycardia, meningitis, retinitis, and paralysis. And the number of "sudden deaths" during and after the pandemic was remarkable.[70]

Encephalopathy or encephalitis—brain fever—accompanying infection with influenza A, and other viruses, is now a well-recognized, if still controversial, phenomenon.[71] The disorder is sometimes referred to as post-viral fatigue syndrome or chronic fatigue syndrome.[72] In 1918 an extraordinary number of cases of encephalitis occurred. The encephalitis seemed to be a new and separate disease first described by a Viennese physician named Constantin von Economo in 1917. The new encephalitis became uncommonly prevalent in England and France in the late winter of 1918, after the worst wave of the pandemic had subsided. The English thought at first that the new "nervous disease," characterized by paralysis of the facial muscles, including those of the eye, might be a result of botulism: food poisoning from spoiled canned food.[73] More striking than the paralytic symptoms, however, was an overwhelming lethargy, a remarkable drowsiness. This sleepiness was such a constant symptom that doctors called the disease "lethargic encephalitis." Cases of the so-called sleepy sickness appeared in the United States in early 1919. Between 1919 and 1923 many hundreds, perhaps thousands, of cases occurred across the country. In 1924 the new encephalitis reached epidemic proportions in Japan, where four thousand of the seven thousand victims died.[74]

Within a year or so after the new disease put in its appearance, the name lethargic encephalitis seemed a misnomer. Some patients were not lethargic at all. They were hyperkinetic instead of hypokinetic, that is, they had increased muscular activity in the form of tics, twitching, and spasmodic, involuntary movements of their limbs or facial muscles.[75] Still another group of patients suffered from a third form of the disease—hiccoughs lasting for days. Consequently, doctors decided that "epidemic encephalitis" might be a more appropriate name to describe the strange disease.[76]

In the 1920s, Dr. Simon Flexner, Director of the Rockefeller Institute for Medical Research, developed a special interest in epidemic encephalitis, particularly its possible connection with influenza. Flexner believed that epidemic encephalitis was a serious disease because of its after-effects. While the paralyzed muscles of the face tended to improve with the passage of time, those elsewhere in the body did not. Sometimes there were marked mental changes in the victim, changes capable of altering the personality, or resulting in the syndrome known as Parkinson's disease, *paralysis agitans*. Furthermore, Flexner thought that many insubordinate and recalcitrant children and young offenders against the law had been victims of epidemic encephalitis, "from which recovery has been seeming and partial only."[77] Recent reports in the literature have shown that post-influenza encephalitis occurs frequently in children and young adolescents, and it has been postulated that this is a consequence of their less mature immune system.[78] It could also be speculated that the damage caused to the immune system by the vicious attack of the influenza virus would render the central

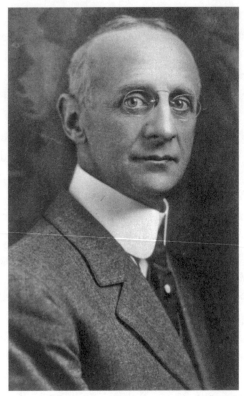

4. Simon Flexner, M.D.

nervous system more vulnerable, possibly by residual dysregulation of the production of inflammatory substances.

The Rockefeller director came to the conclusion, over the course of a number of years, that influenza and epidemic encephalitis were unconnected viral diseases.[79] It had been mere coincidence that they had erupted at the same time, at the end of the war. In the 1970s, however, scientific investigators postulated a link between influenza virus infection and post-encephalitic parkinsonism. Parkinsonism appeared in about eighty percent of those suffering from epidemic encephalitis in the post World War I years. Immunofluorescent techniques appeared to demonstrate the presence of influenza virus antigen in post-encephalitic parkinsonian brains. The viral antigen was not found in the brain of those suffering from idiopathic parkinsonism.[80] Such findings suggested that the two types of parkinsonism might have different etiologies. This theory was supported by the fact that post-encephalitic parkinsonism was a disease rarely encountered any longer, while idiopathic parkinsonism was as common as ever. The findings suggested that some pandemics may cause more brain damage, and that some influenza strains may possess more virulence—more toxicity—than others.

More recently, molecular analysis of well-preserved archival brain tissue from encephalitis lethargica, or post-encephalitic Parkinson cases, has not detected the presence of viral RNA.[81] The analyses were conducted independently in the United States and the United Kingdom, and the conclusions of these groups were that either a link was unlikely—or if there were a link—the virus was no longer present in the brain at the time of death. Like many other aspects of the 1918 pandemic, this question still has no satisfactory answer.

Yet another aspect of the riddle of influenza is why "swine flu" appeared as if it were a new disease during the major wave of the 1918-20 pandemic. First reported by Iowa veterinarian J.S. Koen, the disease affected millions of swine in the autumn of 1918.[82] Although Koen apparently thought that swine caught influenza from humans, the disease became known as swine influenza or "hog flu."[83]

Many other animal species had influenza in 1918. Equine influenza, in fact, had been a serious problem for the military all through the war, even before the human pandemic began. In the fall of 1918 reports came from Africa that scores of baboons were dying from the pandemic disease, and from Northern Canada that influenza was "decimating the big game." At Yellowstone National Park many of the bison, elk, and other animals became ill with the disease, and some died.[84]

Type A influenza viruses are recoverable, in fact, from several domestic and wild animal species, and from birds as well.

Scientists have discovered more than one hundred Type A variants among the birds. Interestingly enough, the first influenza virus to be discovered was a non-human strain. In 1931, two years before the British research team isolated the first human Type A virus, an American scientist, Richard E. Shope, isolated a Type A virus from swine ill with influenza.[85]

Following Shope's work on hog flu, positive evidence that Type A viruses could infect other animals came in 1956. In that year a Type A virus caused an epidemic among the horse population in Czechoslovakia. Seven years later a second Type A virus pathogenic for horses was found in the United States.[86]

At first, flu viruses seemed to be species specific. But the early studies on the potential infectivity of animal viruses for humans were based only on the (H) antigen. Studies made after the discovery of the (N) antigen revealed that several species of birds shared the same (N) antigens with humans. More recently scientists have learned that human influenza viruses are pathogenic for many animals—dogs, cats, chickens, calves, and bears. Thus, the belief that many animals had influenza in 1918 seems to have some basis.[87]

There has also been a continued interest in and curiosity about swine influenza because the disease erupts among the swine population every autumn. Some virologists therefore believe that the virus discovered in 1931 was probably the same one that affected swine in 1918, and that it may have been antigenically related to the 1918 human pandemic strain. This theory was confirmed by a study in 1935, of humans in London, England, who had lived through the 1918 pandemic but had probably never been in contact with swine. Blood samples from the group indicated the presence of antibodies which recognized the 1918 swine virus.[88] Because that swine strain seemed to have been in circulation since 1918, some scientists later suggested that animal reservoirs of infection may exist; that old strains probably never disappeared, but remained viable in some non-human species, potentially capable of combining with some circulating human strain.[89] Interspecies combinations have since been found to occur under natural conditions, and indeed some of the more virulent strains, such as the 1918 variety, are thought to be the result of interspecies recombinations.[90] As such, it is possible that a deadly pandemic could occur at any time, produced by a chance combination of interspecies viral antigens in some unsuspecting individual anywhere on our planet. Such a situation could arise, for instance, if a human suffering from a currently circulating human strain of influenza were living or working in close proximity to swine infected with a swine strain.

When the 1957 pandemic, which appeared to start in Kweichow, China, and then became global within a year, erupted, there was renewed interest in the old theory that influenza pandemics were a product of the Far East. At that time, in many areas of the Far East, humans, pigs and birds (another well-recognized reservoir of influenza strains), often lived in close proximity to each other, as they still do to this day. The World Health Organization consequently encouraged attempts to find the possible existence of an animal reservoir in Central Asian swine. At least one distinguished virologist, however, thought that "the idea of the influenza virus lurking in some remote Mongolian pigsty and bursting out from time to time is an entertaining one, but will scarcely bear critical examination."[91] He and other skeptics cited 1918 as an example of pandemics arising from multiple foci.[92] But when the next pandemic began in Hong Kong in July of 1968, the theory of a Far Eastern origin—human or animal—received more support.

What, then, was noteworthy about the pandemic of 1918? First, it frightened people because no one knew its cause or how it related to pneumonia. Second, it took the American nation and much of the world by surprise because wartime conditions helped to keep its presence a secret for months. Third, about fifty percent of the deaths were among people aged twenty to forty. Fourth, many victims of the 1918 pandemic had long sieges of illness and serious after-effects. Finally, the 1918 strain of influenza apparently affected non-human species as well.

Some medical scientists today think that the recurrence of another pandemic with so many fatalities, reportedly between 50 and 100 million in 1918, is highly unlikely. The basis for such optimism is the belief that many of the pandemic-related deaths in 1918 were the result of secondary bacterial infections. Such bacterial infections could be prevented or controlled today by the administration of antibiotics.[93]

Yet some of the pathologists who did the autopsies on soldier after soldier or on one pregnant woman after another in the fall of 1918 thought that the bronchopneumonia they were finding was not bacterial in nature. Just how many victims the influenza virus did kill in 1918 will remain a mystery. The age-old prescription is still valid: go to bed, keep warm, take aspirin to keep down the fever and drink plenty of liquids. Then, with luck, the infection will clear up in a few days.[94]

In conclusion, influenza is hardly a minor disease. When new pandemic strains emerge, much of the nation (and world) goes to bed. National economics are temporarily affected, and classrooms empty. The social, political, and economic repercussions of epidemic disease may indeed be far-ranging. The next chapter highlights how influenza became a "silent foe" across America during the spring of 1918. Wartime conditions had already contributed to an increase in respiratory infections, and physicians were unaware that the grave pneumonia problem was being compounded by the new pandemic virus. Even when "Spanish flu" took on global significance in the late spring and summer that year, Americans dismissed it as a European disease. Only when millions of people at home, in and out of military service, fell almost simultaneously under the impact of the virus in the early fall of 1918, did influenza become recognized as the nation's prime public health problem.

2

The Silent Foe (Spring 1918)

In the fall of 1917, enroute to Camiers, France, Dr. Harvey Cushing wrote in his diary: "All the world has a coryza."[1] And so it seemed to many observers for the next year or two. One of Cushing's fellow-Bostonians, Dr. Joseph Aub, who was serving in the Massachusetts General Hospital unit in France that fall, recalled nearly forty years later that the pneumonia-flu epidemic of World War I lasted for almost a year. He dated the onset as beginning at Christmas-time 1917, when seventy-five pneumonia victims were admitted to his hospital and became his charges. The mortality rate for that group was a shocking seventy-five percent, a figure, one might suspect, that was probably, at least partially, the result of battlefield conditions in France.[2] At the same time, however, in the military establishments in America, pneumonia, together with a multiplicity of other infectious diseases, was creating large-scale problems for the Army's medical experts and for the Secretary of War, Newton D. Baker.

One historian of the 1918 influenza pandemic has suggested that prior to its onset, disease had had no effect on America's politics and economy.[3] This was hardly true, at least as far as politics was concerned. The First World War had begun in 1914, and it had been a brutal campaign. President Woodrow Wilson had, since then, resisted immense pressure to lead the United States into the

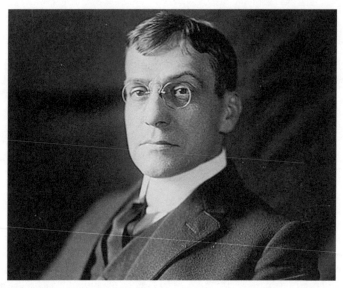

5. Secretary of War Newton D. Baker

War, but when he finally did in April 1917, he did so with complete commitment, sending hundreds of thousands of men first to the training camps and then to the front lines. By the time the American Expeditionary Force (A.E.F.) began to arrive in Europe, the allies were facing a sustained offensive in France from the overwhelming number of German troops at the Western Front, and the French Premier Georges Clemenceau was appealing to the Americans to *come quickly*.[4] During the early months of mobilization, which began about September 1917, the incidence of disease, particularly measles, in the camps rose sharply. "Death Invades Camps" became an all-too-frequent front-page caption in the nation's newspapers. The United States Army had grown at an explosive rate, from a few tens of thousands of men before the war to millions within a few months. Such growth posed an enormous challenge for those responsible for providing their accommodation—a challenge that was not met with great success.[5] Before the winter of 1917-18 had ended, the demand for Secretary Baker's resignation was frequently heard, particularly from the Republican minority in Congress.[6]

With off-year elections to follow in the fall, and Party advantage hard to come by because of the bipartisan support given the war effort, politics and disease became intimate bedfellows during the winter of 1917-18.

In January 1918, the "father of military preparedness," former Congressman Augustus Peabody Gardner of Massachusetts, then Major Gardner, caught cold at a rifle range at Camp Wheeler, Georgia. Within only a few days he was dead of pneumonia. The fifty-two year-old politician had been the first congressman to resign his seat to enter the Army. He was also the beloved son-in-law of that inveterate enemy of the Wilson administration, Senator Henry Cabot Lodge. Gardner's death brought a quick response in Washington, where Ohio's Representative Warren Gard, a Democrat, introduced into the House a resolution calling for an immediate congressional investigation of camp and hospital conditions. The *New York Times* made the comment that although Gardner's premature death from pneumonia could not be attributed to any fault of the camp's health conditions, it was "a striking coincidence that he succumbed at a time when the country had begun to grumble over defects in Army management due to a lack of the wholehearted preparedness he [Gardner] had advocated."[7]

Much of the criticism of the Democratic administration came to focus upon the War Department. Baker's alleged negligence in providing adequate hospital facilities and medical supplies for the young Army recruits soon became President Wilson's Achilles' heel. The public was in a somber mood in January 1918 when Congress summoned Secretary Baker to appear on the national witness-stand for three days.[8] The congressional military committee investigating the apparently deficient health provisions at the training camps asked Baker to explain why so many men were dying at a time when they were so desperately needed for the war effort. The Secretary probably could not be held directly responsible for the increase in measles and mumps infections, which statistics suggested were closely allied with the mobilization process itself. But the deaths following measles and minor respiratory infections were another matter. Many of these pneumonia deaths were to be laid by Congress and others at Baker's doorstep.

During the early months of 1917, shortly after the United States had entered the war, Secretary Baker had met with a blue-ribbon committee of physicians to analyze the medical and sanitary needs of the projected new Army camps. Under discussion were such matters as adequate ventilation in the barracks, and the amount of floor space to be allocated per soldier. During that same period—in order to guarantee that the nation would have as healthy an army as possible—the physicians had urged the Secretary to see that hospital facilities would receive a construction priority at every campsite. Sick men, after all, were not only ineffective themselves, but required healthy caretakers to look after their needs.[9] Such were lessons that had been learned from all of the wars in history, when often more soldiers died from epidemic disease than on the battlefield or as a result of their wounds, a situation the physicians desperately hoped to avoid.

Despite Secretary Baker's early interest in medical provisions, the Army that began camp life in the fall of 1917 found the camps still under construction, with inadequate sanitary facilities the general rule. Hospitals were too often the last buildings erected. Moreover, as the crisp autumn turned into an unusually frigid winter, the lack of warm uniforms and blankets compounded the problem. Severe epidemics of measles, complicated by pneumonia, claimed the lives of thousands of soldiers in the camps.[10] As the weekly camp death rates from pneumonia mounted, so did criticism of the War Department.

As the winter came on, along with Secretary Baker, the Army Medical Corps came under public scrutiny as well. The Army Surgeon General at the time was William C. Gorgas, noted for having led the highly successful taskforce that had attacked the yellow fever problem in Cuba and the Panama Canal Zone.[11] Gorgas had no intention of allowing his department to accept the blame

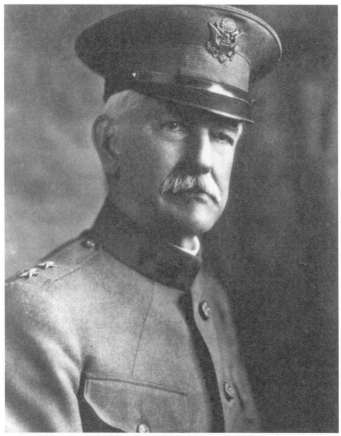

6. Army Surgeon General William C. Gorgas

for the rising mortality rate. He had, even before the construction of the camps began, created a special unit for the prevention of infectious disease, with the very best men assigned to it. That unit was headed by William Henry Welch, a distinguished pathologist and physician who had left his post at Johns Hopkins to advise the Army Surgeon General.[12] When reporters asked Gorgas in December for a summation of the crisis, he placed the responsibility on the War Department. Gorgas told them that he had just returned from inspecting many of the camps and was appalled at the high death rates from pneumonia and meningitis. In many of the camps a lack of warm clothing and overcrowded conditions were contributing to the spread of disease. And, because the War Department had built in haste—apparently more concerned with getting its army off to France than in protecting it from disease—the hospital and other medical facilities were distressingly inadequate.[13] The advice given by the committee of physicians had essentially been completely ignored.

Surgeon General Gorgas also testified before the Senate Military Affairs Committee in late January. Again, he related how the soldiers had been rushed into camps before they were fit for occupancy. Many young Americans, therefore, went to their deaths from disease, as a result of overcrowding and inadequate medical care. Gorgas said that untrained draftees—"country boys"—had been entrusted with the care of the sick in poorly equipped hospitals at the various camps. After the Committee had listened to Gorgas' account of his failure to get hospitals built and provisioned, he offered his opinion that the War Department considered the Medical Department of the Army relatively unimportant.[14]

Gorgas' statements were good news for the opponents of the administration. Senator James Wadsworth of New York observed that "the testimony furnished 'a perfect instance' of the lack of team work and planning which the committee had complained of as characterizing the entire conduct of the war."[15] When Senator Wadsworth suggested near the end of the Surgeon General's testimony that there was a lack of efficiency not only inside the War Department, but also in its relations with other governmental agencies, and that there was no "special power" coordinating the activities of the government in the war, Gorgas answered, "I was never in their confidence, no."[16]

Although the Surgeon General had defended some of the actions of the War Department, his testimony, by and large, was critical of Baker's administrative ability. American soldiers were dying as a result of haste and poor planning. During the course of the proceedings, however, Gorgas had to accept some of the responsibility for the general quality of medical care in the Army. He could not, for example, deny that some of the physicians in the Medical Corps were unfit to practice medicine. They, too, had been processed in haste. When the United States entered the war in April 1917, fewer than a thousand medical officers had been on active duty. By February 23, 1918, there were more than fifteen thousand.[17]

Even before the Senate hearings, the Surgeon General's office had begun to weed out the unfit in the Medical Corps. During this same period—between America's entry into the war and February 23, 1918—where the Army gained so many thousands of additional medical officers, the Corps also dropped more than a thousand medical men.[18] In general, the mustering out had been a quiet one, a departmental matter. When the health of the Army became a political football in the winter of 1917-18, however, alleged cases of gross negligence on the part of medical officers received wide publicity in the nation's newspapers. Letters from distressed and irate parents were forwarded to members of Congress, to Secretary Baker, and sometimes to the President.[19] To assure the public that it would not tolerate gross neglect and misjudgment, the War Department instituted court-martial proceedings against medical officers at Fort Zachary Taylor, near Louisville, Kentucky, and at Camp Doniphan, Fort Sill, Oklahoma.[20]

Despite efforts to improve the quality of medical care, the number of pneumonia deaths remained high. Dr. Victor C. Vaughan, in charge of the Army Medical Corps' division of communicable diseases during the war, later wrote of his department's unfortunate record during that period. The standard the division had hoped to establish was to keep morbidity and mortality statistics in the various camps at a level comparable with those in the civilian sector for the same age group. However, that goal was realized in only a few camps. From September 29, 1917, to March 29, 1918, a period of six months, only five of the twenty-nine major camps succeeded in meeting the standard. During that time the average death rate from pneumonia in the twenty-nine camps was twelve times as great as that in the civilian sector. Dr. Vaughan wrote: "So far did pneumonia overshadow all other diseases that the history of this disease is the medical history of our cantonments."[21]

The Army's pneumonia problem, so apparent by early 1918, had followed in the wake of widespread measles epidemics in late 1917. Every troop train arriving at Camp Wheeler, near Macon, Georgia, in the autumn of that year brought active eruptive cases of measles. Before long there were one hundred to five hundred cases at the camp each day. Of every one thousand soldiers with measles, forty-four developed pneumonia, and of those, fourteen died. The outbreak of measles epidemics in the camps overtaxed the already inadequate medical facilities. These facilities were simply unprepared for hundreds of new patients each day, patients who needed care for almost a month. Isolation techniques proved almost impossible to carry out, and keeping the Army on its feet (or, for that matter, out of the grave) turned out to be a difficult task.[22]

According to Dr. Vaughan, by the end of 1917, the Army's medical personnel had treated 8,479 pneumonia victims. Of those, 952, or 11.2 percent, had died. The worst was still ahead; the seriousness of wartime pneumonia for the Army is indicated in the statistics shown below:[23]

Sept. 29, 1917 – March 29, 1918	April 15, 1918 – August 30, 1918	Autumn 1918 (Pandemic Period)
Pneumonia Cases 13,393	8,912	61,198
Pneumonia Deaths 3,110	1,679	21,053
Case Fatality 23.1 %	18.8 %	34.4%

Even in the late spring and summer months of 1918, when the number of respiratory infections decreased, the percentage of pneumonia victims who died was greater than 11.2 percent during

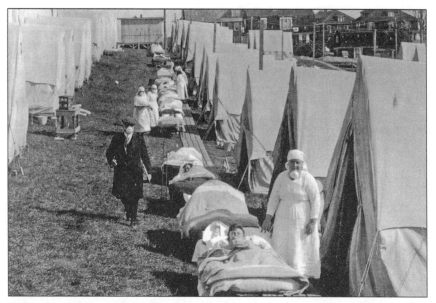

7. Emergency hospital in Brookline, Massachusetts for influenza patients

the so-called period of hasty mobilization of the previous autumn. Despite having better sanitary equipment and additional medical personnel in 1918, the pneumonia problem continued to defy solution, complicated as it was by the arrival of a new pandemic strain of influenza in the early months of 1918.

With the measles epidemic the chief concern of the Army Surgeon General's Office, the mild spring outbreaks of influenza in the Army camps were not the focus of much attention in the early months of 1918. However, many steps were being recommended to minimize the spread of infection, such as the use of separate wards for victims of infectious disease, or at least separate cubicles in hospital wards, and implementing a 10 to 14-day quarantine for new recruits. Whether the Army would be willing to put these in place was another matter.[24]

As the spring of 1918 approached, not only pneumonia but less serious respiratory diseases such as "grippe" and "hard colds" increased in some sections of the country. The civilian population along the Eastern seaboard seemed to have more than its share of grippe. In New York City, the mother of the Assistant Secretary of the Navy, Franklin Delano Roosevelt, elicited concern from her family in February when she came down with a nasty siege of the grippe.[25] A few weeks later Col. Edward M. House, also then in New York, developed a severe case of the grippe as well. The Colonel, President Wilson's trusted and intimate advisor, had to cancel all his engagements and postpone a trip to Washington on March 11 in order to take to his bed. For the next week he cut back on his work schedule, often sleeping until noon, in the hope of getting over his affliction as quickly as possible. When he finally did go to Washington at the end of March, however, the President's physician put him to bed in the White House. Not until the end of April did House believe that he had actually recovered from his respiratory distress.[26]

Some New York residents, less well-known than Mrs. Roosevelt and Colonel House, had fatal respiratory illnesses in March. Early that month seventy-year-old Commodore Jacob W. Miller died after an illness of only two days—the diagnosis: pneumonia.[27] City Magistrate, sixty-one year old Paul Krotel, died of pleuropneumonia and uremic poisoning on March 15, only a few hours after he had consulted a physician. His death occurred a mere two weeks after that of his wife, who had also been a pneumonia victim.[28] But many young people were also dying of respiratory disease. At Camp Upton on Long Island, Lieutenant Gustaf L. Norstedt of the Medical Reserve Corps died of pneumonia on March 16. He was only twenty-six.[29] Two days later, twenty-two year-old Holmes Mallory, a sergeant of the Intelligence Police at Governor's Island, died suddenly at the Hotel Biltmore from a "heart attack following a severe case of the grip."[30] Thirty-three year-old artist, Richard Hamilton Couper, died of pneumonia at the Rockefeller Hospital on March 20.[31] In New Jersey, the president of the sophomore class at Princeton University, Erich M. Enos, died of the same disease the next day.[32]

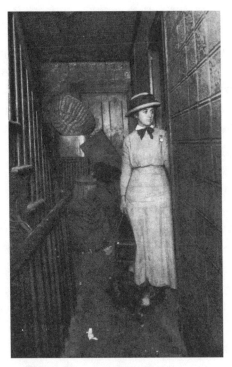

8. A nurse visiting a tenement in New York City

Since most doctors and local and state health departments kept no records of influenza in the spring of 1918, it is difficult to ascertain exactly how widespread the disease was in the New York City area. But some statistics for the presence of pneumonia do exist. The city's overall death rate for January and February of 1918 was actually lower than for the same period in 1917. Despite severe weather, 2,600 fewer people died in the first two months of 1918, and the death rate decreased from 16.97 per thousand in 1917, to 15.51 in 1918. Significantly, the city health report showed a reduction in mortality, with 450 fewer deaths in January and February of 1918 than in the same months of the previous year.[33] In March 1918, however, according to some statistics compiled by Lillian D. Wald's Henry Street Visiting Nurse Service, the city's mortality from pneumonia rose considerably. A record number of calls upon its nursing service were made in March of 1918, resulting from an increase in pneumonia cases. The Visiting Nurses logged five thousand more visits during March 1918 than during the same month in 1917, and the percentage of pneumonia deaths rose from 8.7 in 1917 to 12.3 in 1918.[34] Serious respiratory illnesses were obviously widespread in New York City that March.

One of the few places in the nation to keep a record of influenza cases among the civilian population during the spring of 1918 was the Ford Motor Company in Detroit, Michigan. The company had a medical service for its employees, a benefit then rare in factory life. In March, the Ford medical staff sent 1,066 employees home with influenza. Then, as the month progressed, the number of cases seen each day increased. While only ten cases were seen on March 1, the number of flu victims reporting to the health service on March 27 was fifty-four. The next day the number of new cases almost tripled: 145. For the next ten days Ford's medical service saw an average of 168 influenza sufferers each day. Then the epidemic declined and was apparently over by the eighth of May. Ford medical authorities estimated that the number of workers sent home because of influenza represented only about half of those in the plant affected by the disease. Many flu victims were able to continue their usual routines and those that went home sick remained away an average of only 3.57 days.[35]

The type of influenza circulating in the Detroit area was evidently more serious than the Ford statistics would suggest. The figures presented in Table 2.1, extracted from Selwyn D. Collins, W. H. Frost, Mary Gover, and Edgar Sydenstricker's, *Mortality From Influenza and Pneumonia in 50 Largest Cities of the United States 1910-1929* (1930), indicate that Detroit's death rate from influenza and pneumonia rose sharply in April 1918.[36] (All of the excess monthly death rates presented in Tables 2.1, 2.2, and 2.3 represent a deviation from the median death rate for the corresponding month for the period 1910-1916.)

Table 2.1: Detroit: Excess Monthly Death Rates (Annual Basis) per 100,000 from Influenza and Pneumonia in 1917-20

	Jan.	Feb.	Mar.	Apr.	May	Jun.
1917	+89	+36	+50	+64	+69	+21
1918	+25	+9	-15	+292	-17	-32
1919	+617	+390	+195	+18	-36	-38
1920	+640	+1,497	+101	+96	+51	-9

	July	Aug.	Sep.	Oct.	Nov.	Dec.
1917	+62	+27	+36	+28	+28	+10
1918	+4	-12	-11	+1,351	+793	+679
1919	+6	0	+1	+8	-8	+55
1920	+8	+11	-4	-6	-12	-19

Many other American cities had high death rates from respiratory diseases during the early months of 1918; in fact, some fatality rates rose as early as January. Of the fifty cities studied by Collins, et al, only four—Fall River, Paterson, Los Angeles, and Spokane—went through the first four months of 1918 without some fair increase in the number of fatalities from respiratory diseases. Table 2.2 lists the other forty-six cities in the Collins study, according to the month in which the excess monthly death rates peaked.[37]

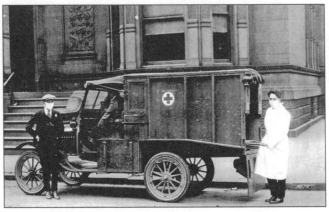

9. Emergency hospital set up in Girl's Club, Philadelphia

Table 2.2: Spring 1918: Months in Which Excess Monthly Death Rates (Annual Basis) per 100,000 from Influenza and Pneumonia Peaked in Forty-Six Cities of the United States

January	February	March	April	April
Wash., D.C.	Boston	Bridgeport	Worcester	Indianapolis
Memphis	Cambridge	New York City	Providence	Chicago
	Lowell	Jersey City	New Haven	Detroit
	Baltimore	Newark	Albany	Grand Rapids
	Richmond	Philadelphia	Buffalo	Milwaukee
	New Orleans	Kansas City	Rochester	Louisville
		Oakland	Syracuse	Nashville
		Portland	Pittsburgh	Birmingham
			Scranton	Minneapolis
			Atlanta	St. Paul
			Cincinnati	Omaha
			Cleveland	St. Louis
			Columbus	Denver
			Dayton	Seattle
			Toledo	San Francisco

Some of the cities listed in Table 2.2 had increased mortality rates for only one month, while others had high rates for two or three months. Table 2.3 illustrates the wide range of excess monthly mortality rates in eight American cities from November 1917 to May 1918.[38]

Table 2.3: Excess Monthly Mortality Rates from Influenza and Pneumonia in Eight United States Cities from November 1917 to May 1918

Washington, D.C.		New York City		Philadelphia		Cambridge	
Nov	-6	Nov	+19	Nov	+66	Nov	-58
Dec	6	Dec	-4	Dec	+109	Dec	-89
Jan	+180	Jan	+36	Jan	+176	Jan	+38
Feb	+113	Feb	+1	Feb	+122	Feb	+242
Mar	+147	Mar	171	Mar	+186	Mar	-29
Apr	+77	Apr	107	Apr	+119	Apr	+97
May	+58	May	-52	May	+57	May	+38

Richmond		Pittsburgh		Albany		Nashville	
Nov	+76	Nov	+171	Nov	-24	Nov	22
Dec	-56	Dec	+238	Dec	+40	Dec	+6
Jan	-87	Jan	+300	Jan	-106	Jan	+144
Feb	+126	Feb	+156	Feb	-21	Feb	08
Mar	-31	Mar	+154	Mar	+4	Mar	13
Apr	-47	Apr	+897	Apr	+97	Apr	28
May	-34	May	+115	May	-69	May	3

The excess monthly mortality rates for Detroit and the other eight cities show that the civilian population had an increased number of respiratory deaths during the spring of 1918. So the pneumonia problem was not confined to the Army. How many of the pneumonia deaths in the cities were related in some way to influenza is impossible to say, but since influenza fatalities are usually the result of pneumonic complications, the mortality statistics for the combined category Influenza-Pneumonia are certainly revealing.

Although morbidity records indicating any generalized epidemic of influenza was in process during the spring of 1918 are lacking, the U.S. Army and U.S. Navy medical records do show that the two service branches had outbreaks of flu throughout early 1918.[39] Naval records indicate that the first epidemic among their personnel broke out on board the U.S.S. *Minneapolis* at the Philadelphia Navy Yard in January. There were twenty-two cases in all, and the disease subsided within two weeks.[40]

In February, 1918, a few large epidemics occurred among U.S. Naval officers and sailors along the Atlantic coast:

	Cases
U.S.S. *Dubuque* at the Navy Yard, New York	1
U.S.S. *Madawaska*, Cruiser and Transport Service	37
U.S.S. *New Jersey*, Atlantic coast	220
U.S.S. *Salem* at the Navy Yard, Boston	30
United States Naval Radio School, Cambridge, MA	350-400

The large epidemic at the Radio School in Cambridge, Massachusetts, correlated with the sudden rise in the excess monthly mortality rate in the city of Cambridge in February. In the same month, several cases of influenza, complicated by pneumonia, occurred among the crew of the U.S.S. *South Dakota* at the Navy Yard in Portsmouth, New Hampshire. A few men on the U.S.S. *Leonidas* at the same navy yard also had attacks of uncomplicated influenza.[41]

In March 1918, further outbreaks of influenza occurred on the eastern seaboard:

	Cases
U.S.S. *Frederick* at the Navy Yard, Portsmouth, NH	147
U.S.S. *St. Louis* at Norfolk, VA	73
U.S.S. *Charleston* at Hampton Roads, VA	55
U.S.S. *Buffalo* at Philadelphia, PA	21

Doctors also reported influenza in epidemic form on two ships of the fleet located in the Chesapeake Bay area.[42]

In April, the U.S. Navy records indicate that influenza was no longer confined to the Atlantic coast:

- U.S.S. *North Carolina* at Norfolk, VA.; 100 cases of mild type.

- U.S.S. *Pensacola* at the Navy Yard, Charleston, SC; mild epidemic.

- U.S.S. *May*, Base 20, Rochefort, France; 25 per cent of the crew suddenly attacked.

- U.S.S. *Oregon* at Mare Island, CA; approximately 450 men, two-thirds of the ship's company, attacked by influenza.

- U.S.S. *Bath*, Hampton Roads, VA.; 38 cases with 1 death.

- United States Naval Training Camp, Gulfport, MS; mild epidemic but higher percentage of complement was attacked than during the fall 1918 epidemic.

- Seventh Regiment, United States Marine Corps, Santiago de Cuba; mild epidemic which spread rapidly; victims showed immunity in the fall.

- United States Submarine Base, San Pedro, CA; a 10-day epidemic following the visit of a Japanese ship whose crew was suffering from the disease.

- United States Naval Training Camp, San Diego, CA; an epidemic following the visit of a Japanese squadron. Nine percent of the complement were attacked, 410 cases. There were pneumonia complications in 12 cases.[43]

The May record was as follows:

Cases

U.S.S. *Dixie*, Queenstown, Ireland; 11 percent of crew attacked 77

U.S.S. *Texas*, with the British Grand Fleet; 2 deaths 80

U.S.S. *Birmingham* at Gibraltar; 10-day epidemic 78

U.S.S. *Chester* at Plymouth, England; 20 percent of the crew
  attacked.. 80

U.S.S. *Nashville*, passage, Gibraltar to Bizerti, Africa;
  47 percent of the crew attacked 91

United States Naval Air Station, Dunkirk, France; 90 percent
  of the complement attacked .... —

United States Naval Air Station, Gujan-Mestras, France;
  40 percent of the complement attacked 72

Influenza epidemics continued to erupt among U.S. Navy crews during June, July, and August of 1918. Most of the summer outbreaks were evidently "mild," with only occasional pneumonic complications, and only a few deaths. Still, influenza epidemics are uncommon in the summer months. 1918 seemed to be an unusual year in that what was ordinarily considered a "winter sickness" became a disease for all seasons, at least throughout the Navy.[44]

The U.S. Army also recorded morbidity statistics for influenza during the spring of 1918. Albert Gitchell, a company cook, at Camp Funston, Kansas, whose illness began on March 11, has sometimes been designated as the Army's first influenza victim in the spring wave of the pandemic.[45] Others date the first victim at Camp Funston, Kansas on March 4.[46] Dr. Rufus Cole of the Rockefeller Institute thought that he and the other members of a Pneumonia Commission assigned to Fort Sam Houston, Texas, had all caught some new upper respiratory infection even earlier that year. Later, in 1922, Cole recalled that every one of the men in his party had fallen ill with an acute illness that had lasted for a few days and, in some cases, had been characterized by a sore throat

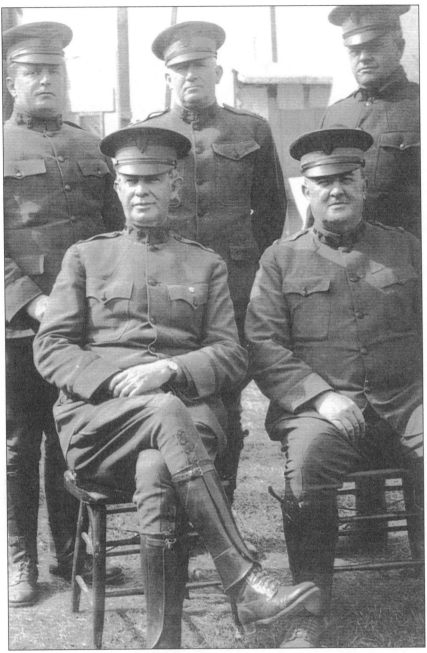

10. Officers in charge of U.S. Army Influenza Hospital, Camp Emery Hill, Lawrence, Massachusetts

or an acute coryza or cough. Because of the serious pneumonia problem at the camp, the investigators had given little thought to this less serious epidemic. But, Cole insisted, there could be little question that an epidemic had been present. It had been "a subject of conversation among the men, and the dust, the weather and especially the occurrence of 'Northers' were all blamed."[47]

The epidemic Dr. Cole described at Fort Sam Houston occurred weeks before Albert Gitchell became a victim of the flu. One of the members of Dr. Cole's Pneumonia Commission, Lieutenant Francis G. Blake, reported for duty at the Texas camp on February 15. Four days later, he wrote home that although he had been perfectly well so far, "All the other men have had or are having 'Texas colds'." The epidemic described by Cole occurred in February of 1918.[48]

Lieutenant Blake, who remained at Fort Sam Houston after the Pneumonia Commission completed its work on March 18, served for a time as an apprentice ward surgeon at the Fort's hospital. Before he left to take up his new assignment as supervisor of the Camp Merritt, New Jersey pneumonia service in early April, he spent most of his time examining flu victims. On March 26 he wrote home, "Have been busy on the ward all day—some interesting cases—gastric ulcer, tuberculosis, etc. But most of it [is] influenza at present."[49] By March Blake and the other physicians tended to diagnose the "Texas colds" as influenza.

But the "Texas colds" in February were not the first instance of respiratory disease approaching epidemic proportions among the military. Camps from California to Virginia had serious outbreaks of respiratory disease all through the winter of 1917-1918.[50]

Table 2.4 indicates the sizable increase in acute respiratory disease in one Army camp during the early months of 1918. Dr. Rufus Cole extracted the figures from the Army Surgeon General's Annual Report for 1919.[51]

Table 2.4: Camp Lewis, Tacoma, Washington: All Acute Respiratory Disease by Month 1917-18; Admission Rate per 1,000

1917		1918	
October	57.11	January	369.73
November	196.81	February	253.06
December	198.36	March	860.62
		April	770.74
		May	337.52
		June	212.76
		July	318.21
		August	261.05
		September	470.26
		October	1,452.54
		November	753.42
		December	763.19

The Camp Lewis statistics indicate how widespread respiratory infections were in the Army during the war. In January 1918 there was a marked increase in respiratory disease, but in March and April greater numbers of troops fell ill. The high admission rates for March and April no doubt reflected the onset of pandemic influenza. Even during July and August of 1918 respiratory disease was a serious problem. The admission rates for those two months were higher than the rate for the previous February. Influenza and pneumonia continued to occur among the Army personnel long after the spring wave of the pandemic had subsided. Whenever a fresh group of susceptible individuals appeared in the camps, there was apt to be another outbreak of respiratory and other infectious diseases.

But the epidemics of influenza at the U.S. Army camps during the spring and summer months of 1918 curiously varied from camp to camp. Considerably more soldiers died from acute respiratory disease at Camp Funston, Kansas and at Camp Dodge, Iowa than at Camp Dix, New Jersey during March, even though all three camps had high admission rates. Admission rates and case fatality rates showed little correlation, although evidently the March epidemics had higher fatality rates than those in April. Perhaps more than one strain of influenza had circulated during the spring of 1918.[52] Such an occurrence would not be a surprise. If a new and virulent strain of influenza were developing, there may have been a series of flare-ups preceding the major pandemic wave, as the virus acquired the changes it needed to become more transmissible and virulent—a more efficient killer.

Fortunately, the civilian sector of the American population avoided the increased incidence of acute respiratory disease occurring in the Army during the late spring and summer of 1918. The monthly excess death rates in the fifty cities studied by Collins, et al, approached the median rate for the period 1910-16. But some epidemics were still erupting in scattered communities across the country in May. One of those broke out in Massachusetts at Amherst College, where the poet Robert Frost was on the faculty. During the middle of May he became sick, and in consequence, wrote to his daughter, Lesley, that he would have to postpone for a few days the visit with her that he had scheduled. The reason, he wrote on the thirteenth, was the "ill health in the head of the family who is in bed at this moment with something the doctor doesn't know what to call because he hasn't been called in to look at me." Frost added that— as near as the doctor could make out by telephone—"it seems to be this here throatal (throtle) epidemic in Amherst."[53] Lesley, a student at Wellesley College, had had a "fresh cold" in April, apparently one of several during the school term, for her worried mother wrote: "It seems to me that you have been sick nearly all the time this year."[54]

During the spring of 1918 people sometimes called the prevailing influenza a "three-day fever," because the average victim was back on his feet in about that length of time. As previously mentioned, the Ford Motor Company statistics showed an absentee rate of approximately three-and-a-half days. When pandemic influenza struck Shanghai in May and June of 1918, the Shanghai *North China Herald* for June 8 described the "mysterious illness currently laying the Chinese low" in the following manner:

> *Ha! Very strange. Ten men sick this office. Plenty man sick Nanking Road. One goldshop anytime 26 man work, now only 8 man, one small boy. Native city have got one shop 30 more man work, now 28 man head go round, body very warm, no can anything....No, no belong dengga fever. Chinaman talk dengga fever 'red fever.' This fever got no red, only head go round, body very warm, no can anything. Some man say plenty fighting Hunanside, any death man throw Yangtze, walkee Shanghai, water no proper....How fashion foreign man no got sick? He no drinka water, drinks beer, whisk', 'quarus....I think no very strong sick—one day body very warm, head go round, no can anything; next day little can something; next day can walkee.*[55]

In general, the spring wave of the pandemic was "no very strong sick." Robert Frost's case was probably an exception, if it were indeed the flu, for he was still ailing in June. Mrs. Frost wrote to Lesley sometime that month that "Papa is gaining a little...though he still coughs very badly and sweats so readily that it is almost impossible for him to exercise enough to sleep well without taking more cold."[56] But compared with the lethal wave in the autumn of 1918, fewer people had developed complications. Many victims had sore throats and fevers, but they tended to recover fairly promptly.

Nonetheless, minor respiratory illnesses were so prevalent in early 1918 that a "National Campaign Against Colds" began in April, on orders of Army Surgeon General Gorgas. The government arranged for a publicity campaign to protect soldiers and sailors against attacks of respiratory illnesses caused by promiscuous coughing, sneezing, and spitting. Weeks went by, and Washington issued a series of slogans urging people to use handkerchiefs when they sneezed or coughed. The slogans appeared in newspapers, magazines, and on posters in restaurants and trolley cars.[57]

Besides the "Keep Fit" slogans circulating in the spring, a rumor spread that a new and virulent plague had recently made its appearance in Europe. Apparently the plague was undermining both Germany's war machine and its home front. As a result, the Germans had postponed their western offensive until the disease had subsided in late March. Only then had the German onslaught begun.[58]

The rumor evidently circulated on both sides of the Atlantic, for in the fall of 1918, as Harvey Cushing grew progressively weaker following his siege of influenza, he wrote in his journal: "So this is the sequence of the grippe. We may perhaps thank it for helping us win the war if it really hit the German Army this hard in February last...."[59] But there is no evidence to support the existence of a virulent epidemic affecting the German nation and its army in February 1918. In fact it was not until April 1918 that many of the German troops complained of the "blitz catarrh."[60] More likely, the proposal that a new variety of influenza struck Germany as early as February 1918 was a piece of Allied propaganda, an attempt to blame the Germans for being both the source of the new strain of influenza and for spreading it throughout the rest of Europe. In the end, it was the Spanish people who received most of the blame for the deadly disease. Variously known in Japan as "wrestler's fever," and in China erroneously as dengue, the name of the new disease changed in Italy as 1918 progressed from "pappataci fever" to "Spanish Grip," then to "summer grip," and finally to pure and simple influenza. Others mistakenly called it "trench fever" or "trench mouth." But the name that finally took hold everywhere, even though the first epidemics in Europe broke out in France, was "Spanish flu," a name with an exotic air that evidently captured the imagination.

A mystery has, in fact, always surrounded the primary outbreak of the pandemic of 1918. It did not originate in Spain, despite its name. In fact, American epidemiologists tend to believe that American soldiers carried the disease to France.[61] Certainly the American Army was on the move in 1918. Fewer than 200,000 troops went across the Atlantic in 1917, but in January and February of the new year nearly 100,000 additional U.S. personnel made the ocean voyage. Then, beginning in March 1918, the number transported rapidly increased:[62]

March	85,710
April	120,072
May	247,714
June	280,434
July	311,359
August	286,375
September	259,670
October	184,063
To Nov. 11	12,124

American soldiers were not the only troops who arrived in Europe in 1917-18. The British continued to recruit throughout their vast empire. Both the British and the French contracted labor battalions in those years in the Far East, mostly from North China and Vietnam. Furthermore, some of the Chinese laborers bound for France were in transit through the United States at the onset of the pandemic.[63]

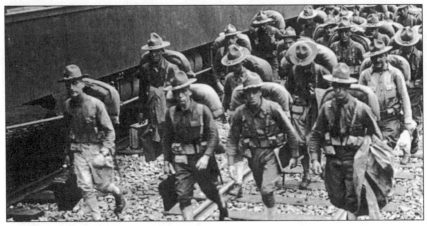

11. The 20th Machine Gun Battalion arrives at Camp Merritt, New Jersey

There is also evidence that suggests that the primary epidemic of the 1918 pandemic might have erupted in the Far East. Therefore, before looking at the condition of the American troops on the transports bound for Europe, it might be worthwhile to investigate what the *Washington Post* first noted on Christmas Day of 1917: "Pneumonia Epidemic in China."

> *Peking, Dec. 24 – There has been a serious outbreak of pneumonia along the Shansi-Mongolia border. More than 100 deaths have already been reported.*[64]

A second report on the situation in China from Tientsin followed on January 6, 1918, in which was noted that the epidemic of pneumonia had reached Fengchengting, in the province of Shansi, 160 miles northwest of Peking, and was causing alarm among the foreigners there.[65] A week later, the *Post* noted that Peking had suspended railroad traffic with the border in order to check the epidemic of pneumonia, and that the government's action had followed upon the demands of the diplomatic corps.[66]

The fourth and final item in the *Post* on the situation in China appeared on January 16 with the caption: "Chinese Threaten American Doctors—Men Sent to Check Epidemic Appeal to be Rescued." According to the short news report, three doctors, two of them American, had gone to Fengchengting to investigate reports of a "plague." There they had been threatened by a mob, which had become angry at their efforts to check the spread of the disease. Consequently, they had sent a telegram to the diplomatic representatives requesting a special train be sent to their rescue. The article went on to relate that "the plague is pneumonic in type," and that although it was spreading in Shansi, the local authorities were indifferent to the encroachment of the disease.[67]

If a serious epidemic of pneumonia *did* erupt in the Far East in the late winter of 1917, why then did it escape the notice of those who searched so diligently for the source of the pandemic?

The answer is that the disease was finally diagnosed as "pneumonic plague," rather than pneumonia or pandemic influenza. But the Chinese malady, first described and tentatively diagnosed by non-medical missionaries as pneumonic plague, was actually shrouded in obscurity. The pneumonia-like disease raged for at least six weeks before health authorities called in the Manchurian plague expert, Dr. Wu Lien-teh. Dr. Wu went to Fengchengting to join the three physicians investigating the plague, and, like them, sought protection against the local inhabitants. Indeed, the riot occurred after Dr. Wu Lien-teh had conducted a few autopsies without first securing permission from the victims' families. It was Dr. Wu who finally made the official pronouncement that the pulmonary disease was "pneumonic plague."[68]

According to the North China Herald, shortly after the riot Dr. Wu stepped down from the supervision of the pulmonary plague because he was ill. A more important reason, however, may have been the dispute over his diagnosis of plague as recounted in a Reuters piece:

> Dr. Ho Shou-yan reports that Dr. Huang and himself have examined the sputum and spleen of two cases reported by Dr. Wu Lien-teh as pneumonic plague. In the first case they found some bacilli, but these were not typical of the bacilli of the pest. In the second case there were no pest bacilli but merely red corpuscles. The bacilli in the first case were quite different from those which Dr. Huang found in 1910 when he was in charge of the bacteriological laboratory of the Sanitary Board in Tientsin, and in his opinion it is doubtful whether these two cases were suffering from pneumonic plague. The Government has consented to permit Dr. Wu Lien-teh, who is suffering from angina pectoris, to return to Peking.[69]

The North China Herald also noted that the majority of the Chinese people also questioned the diagnosis of pneumonic plague.

On January 19, 1918 the same weekly printed the "Chinese Theory" of the situation. Apparently there was a disease known as the "winter sickness" which occurred periodically in the Ordos country in Inner Mongolia. The inhabitants of the area did not regard the illness as anything very remarkable, although it was quite deadly, since a few score deaths evidently occurred from it somewhat frequently. The Chinese seemed to think that the present epidemic was the same, and therefore did not attach much importance to it. Furthermore, the original missionary reports that hundreds were dying had been exaggerated.[70]

Nonetheless, the *North China Herald* noted that three Belgian missionaries had already died of the epidemic disease. It concluded that "whether the 'winter sickness' is identical with pneumonic plague or not, the fact that the missionaries have raised a hue and cry indicates that they regard the present visitation as something quite out of the common."[71]

What made pneumonic plague the logical diagnosis that winter was the widely-held belief that "no other disease than pneumonic plague with even similar symptoms, kills with such rapidity."[72] Many of the victims in North China had died only a day or two after the first signs of illness had appeared. But the disease labeled pneumonic plague, as it progressed in North China, did not always behave in the expected manner. Pneumonic plague was a disease spread by human contact. However, a "peculiar feature" of this particular deadly scourge, noted in Nanking in March 1918, was not only that it was spreading slowly, but there were "only sporadic cases, in some instances connected with each other and in some apparently unconnected."[73] Human contact could not always be traced. Be that as it may, Shanghai officials suggested that people would be safe if they adopted the practice of wearing gauze masks. Those who wore them, however, drew smiles from the Chinese, who referred to the protective devices as "donkey muzzles."[74]

Rather surprisingly, the so-called pneumonic plague simply disappeared in China before the end of April 1918. The coming of milder weather evidently caused its leave-taking. The Shanghai *China Weekly Review* for April 20 reported: "Plague no longer occupies a place in the people's mind. Practically it is forgotten. It no longer exists or appears to exist."[75]

But influenza had now become prevalent in China. In an article written in 1919, S. T. Lee, M.D., a Surgeon Major in the Chinese Army, noted that "last year, 1918, in the months of March, April, and May:

> *There was an extensive epidemic of influenza of the ordinary form without an unusual death rate. This occurred in all the cities along the railways and coast, while in the interior far from the general traffic there were centers of intense infection with pleuropneumonic complications and consequently a very high death rate. At its worst during the months of May and June, the disease was curiously disseminated; two badly infected villages might be separated and between them lie other villages entirely free from the disease or very slightly affected.*[76]

Dr. Lee did add that pneumonic complications were uncommon in the spring of 1918. The purpose of his article, however, was to discourage the belief that the pandemic germ was some variant of the organism responsible for China's "pneumonic plague." He also insisted that China had had both pneumonic plague and influenza in 1917-18, but that its influenza appeared simultaneously with that in France and America, not before. The import of his article was: we have not circulated pneumonic plague—or influenza.

If, however, the Chinese respiratory plague was, in fact, the result of a new pandemic strain of influenza, could it have arrived in the United States and Europe early in the new year? There is evidence that it certainly could have. During the period from July 1, 1917, to June 30, 1918, many thousands of Chinese laborers, transported by the British and French, entered North America at Montreal or Vancouver, traveled by train to an Eastern port (probably New York or Halifax, but possibly Boston), and then set sail on the final leg of their journey for Europe.[77] The laborers were mostly from the Shantung province in North China, the area most affected by the plague in the winter of 1917-18.[78] Thanks to a conscientious diary-keeper, Daryl Klein, a Second Lieutenant in the Chinese Labor Corps, we know that sometime in January— probably before a contingent of two thousand laborers sailed from Tsingtau in the middle of the month—an epidemic was in progress at the labor corps' training camp.[79] He noted: "Many of us are laid up with sore throats, due not only to shouting, but to the dust storms which sweep over the camp at all hours of the day."[80] (Just as in Texas, where they blamed the dust and "Northers".)[81] One of Klein's companions in the camp was a Canadian missionary who, Klein wrote, "has lain sick of a fever for many weeks and who now reappears looking like an alabaster image of a man, as much fit to drill coolies as a delicate nun."[82] Klein also noted in January that their little camp hospital was the busiest of its kind in North China: "Most of the patients are throat or eye or stomach or circumcision cases."[83] Sore throats were fairly common among the laborers as well as the officers.

Besides Klein's observation on the epidemic of sore throats in the camp, a first-hand account in the *North China Herald*, dated Pochow, February 1, 1918 told of a serious plague among cattle and concurrent human throat afflictions:

> My brother has lost six [cattle] in three days, and others are sick. I hear that further south, east of Kuoyang and Mingching they have died in great numbers; also that many people are suffering with a strange throat trouble from which many die about the second or third day after getting it. This may possibly come from their eating the meat of these departed, diseased cows. I heard one man say, rather rejoicingly apparently, that cooked beef is only 30 cash per catty![84]

Strange throat troubles and cattle plague—disease was widespread in China in the winter of 1917-18. If the shipment of Chinese laborers who left Tsingtao in mid-January kept to its schedule, their voyage to Vancouver, via Japan, took approximately three weeks. In another week they might well have been on the east coast of North America. That would have been mid-February, just about the time when the first significant epidemics of influenza began to occur among U.S. Navy personnel stationed along the Atlantic.

The effort to place the primary epidemic in Inner Mongolia in late 1917 is not an attempt to "blame" the Chinese laborers directly for spreading pandemic influenza. The fact is that while the laborers were usually isolated from contact with foreigners on their journey to France, their officers were not. They naturally visited some of the cities that they were passing through.[85] Meanwhile, other American and Chinese diplomatic and commercial traffic was passing freely through customs. Laborers under contract with the French who rode the seas westward, via the Indian Ocean and the Mediterranean, also might have introduced a new viral strain into the port of Marseilles. Vessels from the Orient were making stops at seaports and coaling stations all over the world; they were going around the Cape of Good Hope and through the Panama Canal. Wartime conditions and the shifting of large numbers of workers from place to place virtually guaranteed the rapid spread of pandemic disease.

A number of theories place the origin of the pandemic elsewhere in the world and those are discussed in Chapter 8 of this text. If a new strain of influenza, whatever the origin, arrived in the United States early in 1918 and began to infect the population along the Atlantic coast, then American soldiers probably did carry the virus to England and France. Some may have caught influenza from dockside workers as they left the country, or from naval personnel they might have come in contact with. Despite careful inspection of troops at the eastern ports of embarkation, influenza and other respiratory diseases broke out regularly on the transports. As a result, the voyage to France in the spring of 1918 was, for many troops, a nightmarish experience.

When the U.S.S. *Khiva* sailed from New York on May 20, one of its passengers was Dr. Ira V. Hiscock, the Chief Sanitarian for the U.S. Army's 30th Division Surgeon's Office. On the monotonous journey across the Atlantic, made slower by rough seas, Dr. Hiscock nursed soldiers seriously ill with influenza or P.U.O. (a pyrexia of unknown origin) for almost the entire time. The ship's hospital was full, and when the converted German vessel finally arrived at Liverpool, some of the sick went to hospitals in England. Those who were deemed fit to finish the journey to France went directly to Calais, where still others fell sick. Among them, Dr. Hiscock.

Thus it was that when the 30th Division left Calais, Dr. Hiscock was not with it. Shortly after arriving at the French port, he found himself on a stretcher, on his way to a British hospital somewhere between St. Omer and Cambrai, where he was in bed for about ten days. The Scottish sisters who nursed him back to health had a particular habit he never forgot: each day a sister came around with a dose of castor oil, using the same utensil for patient after patient. Nonetheless, he recovered enough to convince the hospital authorities to release him. After getting out, he hitchhiked to Belgium and prepared to join his division. When he got there, however, he found the division had replaced him with another sanitarian. Evidently the word had circulated that he had been a victim of pneumonia and not the less serious P.U.O. Following some last-minute maneuvering, he managed to march out with his outfit as it left for the Western Front.[86]

But—in the spring of 1918—many American troops found parts of Europe were already under the sway of a new disease, sometimes identified as influenza. Influenza and pneumonia had been common ailments in all of the armies in Western Europe during the winter of 1917-18. One of the flu victims in February

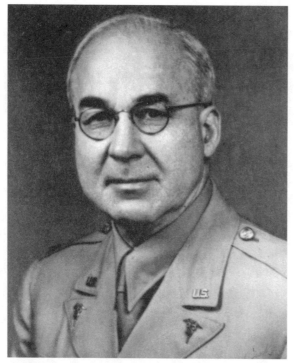

12. Ira V. Hiscock, M.D.

had been an American nurse in Harvey Cushing's Harvard unit. Like the doctor, she kept a diary. The first entry she made was on February 8, 1918, while she lay in a sick bed herself, recuperating from "flu and trench fever." Although she enjoyed the chance to get some much-needed rest, she was anxious to get back to her own hospital so that she would be on hand for the start of the spring offensive. By the middle of February she was back on duty with the Harvard unit.[87]

The Harvard unit, it might be mentioned, was the second of six special medical units organized during the spring of 1917 to work with the British Expeditionary Force.[88] Some of the American medical personnel who went to Europe in May of 1917, Harvey Cushing, for example, did transfer to the U.S. Army's Medical Corps before the war ended. But many of the doctors and nurses served the

British Army until November 11, 1918. The Massachusetts General Hospital nurse, referred to above, was one of the latter. She also was a flu victim again in April 1918. Here is what she wrote in her diary April 23:

> *I am back on my day duty again, working on Bl. And how my back does ache! There seems to be gaps in my writing, but it can't be helped. We've been awfully busy, and besides, I feel beastly. The flu is back again and everybody has it, including me. I've run a temperature of 102 for three days, can hardly breathe, and have to sleep on four pillows at night. But I'm not talking about it, because I don't want to be sent to Villa Tino [a nurses' convalescent home]. Kitty thinks I have a cold on my chest—not knowing about the temperature—though I think she suspected something last night, when I sat up in bed till four in the morning, breathing asthmatically.*[89]

Whether or not she actually had a second case of flu in two months' time may be questioned. If, however, the April 1918 epidemic was the result of the new pandemic strain, she may well have had influenza in February and again in April. The point is that flu was epidemic on the Continent in April as well as in the United States. Only it was not always recognized—or admitted as being Influenza—by nations in the midst of war.

The American public gradually learned of the existence of the new, mysterious ailment during April, May, and June of 1918. Towards the end of April, the captain and crew of an Italian liner, the *D'Abruzzi*, berthed in a slip at the 12th Street pier at Hoboken, New Jersey, only to be struck suddenly by a puzzling illness that resulted in the hospitalization of the captain and sixteen of the thirty-two affected crewmen. The tentative diagnosis was "typhoid fever." However, according to the *New York Times*, some people were quickly jumping to the conclusion that the trouble was the result of "German plotting." In any event, the ship would be quarantined until serologic testing could be completed. A few days later, the paper announced that the tests conducted by the local health authorities found no evidence to indicate the presence of any poison plot. The doctors at the hospitals caring for the affected men had decided they were probably suffering from the "grippe." Nevertheless, government officials were running some special blood cultures to be sure.[90]

By June 1918, newspapers were reporting outbreaks of strange epidemics all over the world. On June 1, the *New York Times* mentioned the mysterious "no very strong sick" in Shanghai. According to the *Times* account, a curious epidemic resembling influenza was sweeping North China.[91] Less than a week later, the same paper noted the "mysterious sickness similar to that in Spain had shown itself in Copenhagen," and that some women were "dropping in the streets by reason of being underfed."[92]

American readers then learned of a new disease called "trench mouth" afflicting British and French troops on the battlefield. The Allied authorities were blaming the German Army for its spread, and suggesting that the root cause was their poor diet of war bread and canned foods. It was true that the diet of the German Army in the summer of 1918 was seldom very healthful. One German diarist complained of having to eat bread as damp as a bath-sponge, and green potatoes dug up well before their harvest time.[93] But while trench mouth was no doubt present in some of the European armies, many of the "red mouths" in the summer were diagnosed in error. They were the mouths of influenza victims, not the result of poor diet or oral hygiene.

Then the Americans learned of wide-scale internal dissension within the German and Austro-Hungarian Empires. June 1918 found Vienna racked by bread riots and strikes. Americans were told "German Hunger Spreads Disease." And, in a special cable from The Hague, they read: "The mysterious sickness now prevalent in Spain comes from Germany and will doubtless soon reach other countries."[94] According to the wire, a Dutch tailor who had recently returned from Germany had found conditions among the civil population there terrible, as he contended that workmen were dying at their tasks from lack of nourishment. Readers were also informed that a widespread wave of disease was decimating Rumania's population.[95]

On June 27, 1918 the *New York Times* centered on page one a two-column spread with the caption: "Spanish Influenza is Raging in the German Army; Grip and Typhus Also Prevalent Among Soldiers." The Germans were constructing special hospitals in the rear areas to deal solely with the new disease. The *Times* caption, incidentally, pointed out the confusion concerning influenza and "grip." The writer of the report apparently thought that they were two separate maladies.[96]

With so many reports of disease circulating in Europe, the War Department thought the time had come to assure the American people that the doughboys were a healthy lot. Consequently, at the end of June 1918 the Department released the following statement:

"No Influenza in Our Army"

Washington, June 27 – No advices have reached the War Department about the influenza among the German troops on the Western front.

The reported epidemic is not regarded here as having serious proportions. It is clear that the soldier who has it is incapacitated for duty, and thousands may be down with the disease at once, so that military movements may be delayed.

The American troops have at no time shown any form of the disease. Precautions have already been ordered, however, to meet any emergency.[97]

This statement was an out-and-out lie, but the deception was designed to allay the fears of parents and relatives of American troops. Meanwhile, Dr. Cole from the Roosevelt Institute and Army Surgeon General Gorgas were trying to get hold of "accurate information concerning the influenza prevailing in Europe." Each had received a number of very worrying reports describing influenza outbreaks of unusual virulence in both America and Europe. The victims of the influenza were dying within 24 to 48 hours, and the mortality rates were alarming, especially among healthy young adults. Members of the pneumonia commission were dispersed around the camps to monitor the disease.

Late in June 1918, the head of the United States Public Health Service (USPHS), Surgeon General Rupert Blue, still did not insist on quarantine for the crew of ships like the British freighter, *City of Exeter*, which arrived in Philadelphia with influenza cases "in a desperate condition" on board. The British consul had himself arranged for the necessary precautions to be taken so that the victims could be disembarked safely and transferred directly to an isolation unit in Pennsylvania Hospital.[98] It was not until early in July that the USPHS finally began to acknowledge there was a problem. Americans learned that passengers arriving on a Spanish ship had been fumigated before the health officers would allow them to leave the vessel. In addition, their clothing had been put through a steamer, lest they contain "some of the germs of the influenza which has been prevalent in Spain for five months."[99] Next, Americans learned that Germans with fever were dropping in their tracks, and that the new disease was getting more serious. It was no longer a "three-day fever." Patients were now being kept in German hospitals for at least *six* days. Possibly the virus grew more virulent as the summer wore on, but the statement had much propaganda value as well.[100] Some American newspapers printed an excerpt from an unposted letter found in the pocket of a German captive on July 4, wherein he discussed the epidemic disease:

I feel so ill that I should like to report sick. Fever is rampant among us and already a whole lot of men are in the hospital. Every day more go in. As I have not yet had leave and am expected to any day, I shall not report sick yet anyway.[101]

Early in July the Kaiser, followed by several members of the German Royal Family, fell ill with influenza.[102] Next came news of Marshal von Hindenburg's undiagnosed illness.[103] Many correspondents thereafter blamed the disease affecting the German civil and military population as being caused by starvation. For example, according to the *New York Times*, July 14, 1918, "The illness from which thousands of persons in German industrial districts are suffering and which has been described as Spanish Influenza is really an illness due to hunger and consequent exhaustion...."[104] The implication was, of course, that the disease would never erupt in the United States. The same paper, on July 26, reported that epidemics were sweeping Germany: "Typhus in Berlin, Malaria in Baden, Influenza Everywhere." It was reported that large numbers of deaths were occurring in the Great Charité Hospital in Berlin and that the health of the enemy's troops had been seriously undermined by the epidemic, with many deaths occurring daily.[105]

Thus as July 1918 ended, the average American knew little about Spanish influenza. So far, he believed, it had not affected his countrymen. He was quite unaware that many of his fellow Americans had already been ill during the spring and that the nation's death rate had been considerably above normal. Influenza had truly been a silent foe for months. Americans believed that they were the best-fed nation, and, in consequence, the healthiest in the world. They were about to win the War for Democracy. Full speed ahead!

But the nation was in for a rude jolt. Over the course of the next five or six months, the so-called European disease would become a universal problem. Not only war, but disease would be global. America would have to mobilize its public health agencies and fight respiratory disease as well as enemy troops. A newly appointed Pneumonia Commission would be thoroughly perplexed by the connection between the pneumonia and influenza cases. Cities like Washington, D.C., which were filled with large numbers of non-resident war-workers, would be especially hard-pressed to cope effectively with the pandemic. Hundreds of thousands of Americans would be dead before November 1918 would come around.

November would bring an end to the war in Europe. But death would continue to claim the lives of thousands of young men and women well after the Armistice.

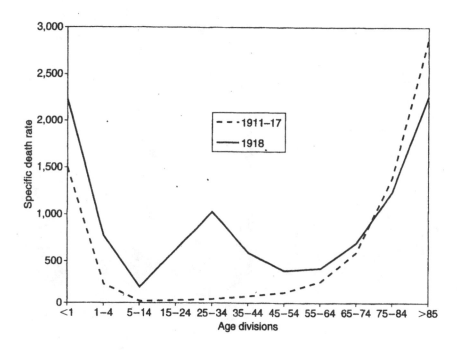

Figure 2.1: Influenza and pneumonia mortality by age, United States. 1918 influenza pandemic year (solid line); average of 1911-15 interpandemic years (dashed line). Death rate is per 100,000 population for each age division.

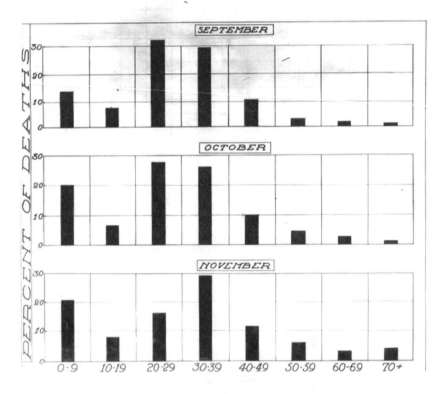

Figure 2.2: Age distribution of influenza and pneumonia deaths at Boston, September-November, 1918.

3

A Kind of Plague (Fall 1918)

"Keep well, my darling, for these are perilous times."[1]

August 1918 began with sickness "over there"—across both oceans. As the month opened, Dr. Peter K. Olitsky of the Rockefeller Institute, who in April had been sent at the request of the British government to help the Hong Kong health authorities with an epidemic of meningitis, was on board the S.S. *Venezuela* returning to America. He had been sick on and off since early July, first with a self-diagnosed severe cold, then influenza, and finally dengue. He arrived home in New York on August 20, recovered from the so-called dengue, but with a serious boil (the second within three months) causing him much pain.[2]

On the other side of the world, James Kerney, director of the Paris office of the American Committee on Public Information, wrote home on August 7 to his long-time friend, Joseph Tumulty, Secretary to President Wilson, relating tales of the Germans' renewed long-distance bombardment of the French capital, and of his impressions of the various French leaders. At the end of the letter, he added: "I've had grip now for about three weeks; it seems impossible to shake it off once it hits you here. Don't mention it to my family."[3]

In his Neufchâteau quarters, just one day before Kerney wrote the above, Dr. Harvey Cushing was recording in his journal that he was resuming his writing "after three days in bed with a N.Y.D. [not yet diagnosed] malady which I regarded as the Spanish flu—three days' grippe—or what you will."[4] The next day he was up and about, but feeling very feeble.[5] The feebleness was so noticeable to his superiors that they ordered him to take a vacation, which he did, passing the following week in Paris, restless with fever, and sleeping most of the time. When he returned to Neufchâteau he was still a sick man, too sick to walk back and forth to his room for lunch. In consequence he resorted to carrying his noon meal in a haversack and eating in his office. As if that were not enough, the muscles of his eyes began to play tricks on him. On September 1 he wrote that he would be wearing glasses henceforth.[6]

Meanwhile, the enemies of the Allies were suffering in like manner. German officer Rudolf Binding, an aide-de-camp to Archduke Charles' Army Group, wrote in his diary on August 12 that he had been having extraordinary attacks of fever, with such general neuralgia that he could "only manage to exist with the help of aspirin and pyramidon."[7]

Binding then came down with a second malady, which he described as a "nasty attack of champagne fever, something like typhoid, with ghastly symptoms of intestinal poisoning." The attack forced him into bed. Five days later he wrote: "I am in the grip of the fever. Some days I am quite free; then again a weakness overcomes me so that I can barely drag myself in a cold perspiration on to my bed and blankets. Then pain, so that I don't know whether I am alive or dead." This, he wrote, had been going on for weeks.[8] He was finally admitted with a bad case of dysentery to the Reserve Hospital at Baden Baden. Neither Cushing nor Binding fully recovered from their summer illnesses by November 11, 1918. Each had to listen to the sounds of the Armistice celebrations through sickroom windows.

Dual attacks of illness like Binding's were common in each

of the antagonists' camps during the summer of 1918. Besides continued flare-ups of influenza, epidemic diarrhea (or dysentery) appeared so often as to cause serious difficulties and excessive sick rates. Immediately after the Chateau-Thierry offensive in mid-July, about seventy percent of the American troops were over the course of two or three weeks somewhat incapacitated by diarrhea. Many of them managed to recover without the aid of medical assistance. Nevertheless, the disease persisted throughout the A.E.F. from July 1 through the middle of September, when it was succeeded by the more deadly wave of influenza. Neither side had healthy armies during the summer, with the two diseases—influenza and dysentery—debilitating thousands every week.[9]

During August, numerous outbreaks of influenza were also occurring among the crews and passengers of vessels returning to the United States from Europe. The *Bergensfjord*, arriving on the twelfth, had two hundred cases of flu, with five deaths, during her return voyage from France, while lesser epidemics broke out on the *Rochambeau* and the *Nieuw Amsterdam*.[10] In the same period a steamship arrived at Newport News with virtually the entire crew affected.[11] Arriving in the United States on the *Espagne* in the latter part of that month was John Dos Passos, who lamented the death at sea of a charming little Swiss woman whom he had befriended on the ship. Of her husband, Dos Passos wrote in his diary: "Poor little man landing in New York with his wife's body—what a hell."[12] Later when he wrote *Nineteen Nineteen*, the second volume of *U.S.A.*, he would record her death for posterity in his unpunctuated prose: "when the immigration officer came for her passport he couldn't send her to Ellis Island la grippe espagnole she was dead."[13]

Despite the increasing numbers of in-bound travelers suffering from influenza during the summer, the U.S. Public Health Service refused to mandate a general quarantine on all incoming vessels. The Service did send out a cautionary letter, however, suggesting that the medical officers in charge of each quarantine station be on the alert for cases of the so-called Spanish influenza.[14]

Any vessel with flu on board was to be held in quarantine until local health authorities had been notified and fumigation procedures set in motion. The circular also noted that the disease appeared to be an infection due to B. Influenza with predilection to lung involvement. However, the circular ended with the following words: "This circular does not contemplate consideration of cases of ordinary pneumonia or respiratory infections, but only those infections involving a considerable number of the crew and which appear to be highly communicable and suggestive of epidemic influenza."[15] Just how the local medical officer was to determine what an ordinary case of pneumonia was, the circular did not say.

In New York City, that port's health officer told reporters in mid-August that there was not the slightest danger of an influenza epidemic breaking out in New York and that he did not plan to adopt quarantine measures.[16] City health officials, however, were a little more wary and decided to order a "watch on ship passengers who have the disease."[17] Although the Chief Surgeon of the New York port of embarkation, Colonel J. M. Kennedy, M.C., U. S. Army, soon assured reporters that the new disease was not at all dangerous, except when pneumonia developed, many passengers who had been victims of the new influenza either in Europe or on the journey to America thought it more malignant, leaving one's system weaker than the common garden variety of flu did. According to one sufferer, "It gives its victims a bad headache and a worse grouch."[18]

On August 5 the Red Cross's weekly bulletin made note of the rising incidence of influenza in Switzerland and other parts of Europe. The bulletin reported that the Surgeon General's office was awaiting information from abroad, supplementary to the special cables that had already been received, to determine whether it was a new disease or simply the well-known form of influenza, with an increased virulence. In the meantime, the Red Cross War Fund had appropriated $125,000 to assist the government of Switzerland to deal with the epidemic of Spanish grippe that had already assumed such alarming proportions in that country.[19]

Two weeks later, on August 19, the *New York Times* made its first admission that United States troops were suffering from influenza: "A considerable number of American negroes, who have gone to France on horse transports, have contracted Spanish influenza on shore and died in the French hospitals of pneumonia."[20] Here in this country pneumonia was increasing among the military. The Army's death rate from respiratory diseases had reached its 1918 low in June. During July the death rate had climbed only slightly, but as August progressed each week the rate rose higher.[21]

All through the spring of 1918 there had been a demonstrable need to appoint a permanent Pneumonia Commission to investigate and carry out laboratory studies on the organisms causing the respiratory deaths at the training camps. When the pneumonia fatalities had begun to increase in late 1917, the Army Surgeon General's office had appointed a few temporary commissions, often with civilians from the Rockefeller Institute, which after all, had few peers when it came to research on pneumonia. But the availability of Rockefeller scientists disappeared early in 1918 when the Institute gave up its civilian status to become U.S. Army Auxiliary Laboratory No. 1.[22] Its staff, with few exceptions, became commissioned officers assigned to teach the Army Medical Corps the latest approaches to scientific medicine and vaccine therapy.

The other paramount medical institution in the nation, Baltimore's Johns Hopkins, was also army-oriented during the war. The dean of the Hopkins' medical community, Dr. William H. Welch, occupied a desk in Surgeon General Gorgas' office, and Johns Hopkins provided so many of the top-level physicians in the A.E.F. that some of the other medical centers must have felt a twinge of resentment. As Dr. Cushing wrote: "Looks a good deal like a transplanted Johns Hopkins, but after all the thing to do is to get the best men and let people criticize if they wish."[23] Johns Hopkins also sent a medical unit, including thirty-two medical students, to work with the A.E.F. The Hopkins' Base Hospital No. 18, located at Bazoilles, near the Meuse, soon became known to the

American medical personnel as the "Bacillus on the Mess."[24] With so many of the top medical scientists in Europe or teaching courses at the Rockefeller laboratory center, it was difficult for the Surgeon General's office to find a group of competent pneumonia investigators who were not already carrying out important assignments for the military.

The five men finally appointed to the permanent Pneumonia Commission in late July of 1918 were exceptionally well-qualified to carry out their assignment. They were Majors Allen W. Freeman and Eugene L. Opie, Captain Francis G. Blake, and First Lieutenants Thomas M. Rivers and James C. Small, two of whom—Blake and Rivers—had served on the temporary commission at Fort Sam Houston, Texas under Dr. Cole, during the previous winter. Their new assignment was to start at Camp Funston, Fort Riley, Kansas.[25]

Arriving during the last few days of July the five men quickly became acquainted or reacquainted as they began their pneumonia studies. According to Blake, Opie was an "excellent pathologist," and Freeman a first-rate epidemiologist. The others, Small, Rivers, and himself, would be doing bacteriological and clinical work.[26]

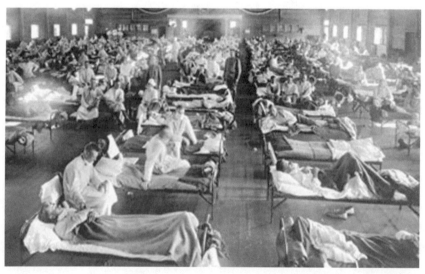

13. Emergency hospital during influenza pandemic at Camp Funston, Kansas

The members of the Commission soon discovered that the pneumonia at the camp was "practically all typical lobar pneumonia due to type pneumococci in about the same proportions that are found in civil life."[27] This was considered pretty dull stuff for the group. And, the "measles streptococcus pneumonia," so common at the Army bases the previous winter, was not present in their patients either. As such, most of their work for the next few weeks concerned newly-arrived Negro draftees from Louisiana and Mississippi. Little or no pneumonia had developed among the ten thousand white troops who had come to the camp in June and July, whereas in a like number of Negro draftees during the same months the rate had been about ten per thousand, a distressingly high incidence. The Commission members thought their bacteriological findings might be significant: "The interesting feature of these cases is that they are practically all types III, IV, and atypical II's." These were the types of pneumococci found in normal throats; consequently the pneumonia in these two groups of men was "due to autogenous infection and not to contact."[28] Although the Commission tended to blame the respiratory infections on the lowered resistance of the men, probably resulting from the after-effects of the draftees' typhoid vaccinations and the changes in the men's physical environment, one might suspect that some of the pneumonias among the Negro troops were viral in nature. Racial segregation could also explain why the pneumonias were occurring almost exclusively in the Negro troops.

Life at Fort Riley, Kansas, in August was soon unbearable. On August 9, Captain Blake wrote home these poignant words:

No letter from my beloved for two days, no cool days, no cool nights, no drinks, no movies, no dances, no club, no pretty women, no shower bath, no poker, no people, no fun, no joy, no nothing save heat and blistering sun and scorching winds and sweat and dust and thirst and long and stifling nights and working all hours and lonesomeness and general hell—that's Fort Riley, Kansas.[29]

Even work did not proceed smoothly. On the morning of August 16, 1918, when Rivers and Blake arrived at the laboratory, they found that the second lot of mice they had injected had all become contaminated "by lying around that hot laboratory during the night so that all that work has gone for nought...."[30] (The previously injected lot had died within twenty-four hours.) And the heat continued unabated. On the wards thermometers had to be passed around in cocktail glasses full of crushed ice, otherwise the temperatures would range from 102 to 106 degrees, depending on the time of day. In the laboratory the investigators had to be certain to keep the incubator door shut, as the outside heat was capable of killing off all of the germs. Captain Blake wrote: "Imagine going into an incubator to get cool."[31]

Happily, travel orders for the Pneumonia Commission arrived from Washington on the thirty-first of August. In the latter part of that month, the camps showing the most pneumonia were Pike in Arkansas, Travis in Texas, and Gordon in Georgia.[32] Although the Commission hoped it might be sent to Camp Gordon, the telegram informed them that their destination would be Camp Pike. By September 5 the doctors were all settled in at the Arkansas post. There, to their amazement, early studies indicated that while pneumonia was not very prevalent, what was there was an entirely new type—"a bronchopneumonia not due to the hemolytic streptococcus at all, but to the influenza bacillus."[33] Blake wrote home on September 12 that Rivers and he had a private hunch that, from the look of things, there was going to be a big influenza bacillus epidemic that year instead of a hemolytic strep as in the previous year—but, of course, they might be wrong.[34] Within another week the members of the Commission found themselves in the midst of an epidemic of influenza and influenzal pneumonia, and the Arkansas newspapers were reporting similar epidemics in Boston and New Orleans. Influenza would probably sweep across the country before winter came.

It might be mentioned that camps other than those under

investigation by the Pneumonia Commission often received visits from the "brass" in the Surgeon General's office. But as Colonel William H. Welch noted, a visit by Colonel Victor C. Vaughn and himself (the two men had been dubbed the "Gold Dust Twins" by their medical associates on the Council of National Defense) was not a cause for rejoicing.[35] It usually meant the camp had an undue amount of sickness.[36] Sometime around September 4, 1918, Welch and Vaughn, along with their SGO colleagues, Colonels F. F. Russell and R. I. Cole, headed south to make an inspection of Camp Wheeler, near Macon, Georgia, and other Southern camps.[37] While on the tour, at a stopover in Asheville, North Carolina, Colonel Vaughn came down with what he diagnosed as a "severe coryza." He was still suffering upon his return to Washington about the twenty-first, when the Surgeon General ordered the inspecting team to proceed at once to investigate a serious outbreak of influenza at Camp Devens, near Ayer, Massachusetts. All or most of the group who had toured in the South now left for Devens, including the watery-eyed Colonel Vaughn.[38]

By the time the men from Washington arrived in the Boston area to travel to Fort Devens, influenza had reached epidemic proportions in New England, and the rest of the nation soon shared its fate. The first cases in the autumn wave of the disease appeared among U.S. Naval personnel at Commonwealth Pier in Boston on August 27. By early September, influenza had arrived at the U.S. Naval stations in Newport, Rhode Island, and New London, Connecticut. On September 7, the first cases of the disease entered the base hospital at Camp Devens. At the same time, Lowell, Lawrence, Brockton, and other Massachusetts factory towns reported multiple cases of flu. Then, in quick fashion, Rhode Island and Connecticut towns had outbreaks of the new influenza.[39]

At first the epidemic was hardly considered a serious matter. On September 10 a Boston newspaper, upon learning that more than a thousand cases of the disease had occurred among local Navy personnel, playfully suggested that the "Girls of Boston Must Cut

Out That Germy Kiss."[40] At the same time, U.S. Naval stations displayed posters containing the following message:

Avoid the hug,
Avoid the lip,
Escape the bug
That gives the "grippe."[41]

The disease spread rapidly, and such levity disappeared when the obituary columns grew longer throughout the northeast. Towards the end of September, Robert Frost's wife, Elinor, wrote to her daughter, Lesley, who had gone to work in an airplane factory instead of returning to college, that she must not go to see her sister, Irma, a student at Dana Hall, Wellesley, Massachusetts, the following Sunday unless she was absolutely certain that the school was free of influenza. Mrs. Frost was especially concerned that both girls already had colds, so early in the new season. Furthermore, there were seventy-two cases of influenza in Littleton, New Hampshire, near where the elder Frosts were then staying, and Mr. Cummings, the lawyer, had died of it the previous Sunday, leaving behind a critically ill wife. They, Mama and Papa Frost, had not yet returned to the Amherst campus, because the college had postponed its opening for two weeks on account of the influenza.[42] Mrs. Frost had good reason to worry about her children, for the new influenza was doing much more than incapacitating its victims—it was killing scores of them.

The outbreak at Camp Devens escalated rapidly. On the eighteenth, eleven days after the first cases reported sick, over one thousand soldiers were admitted to the hospital. By the time Welch and his men arrived at the camp on September 23, the statistics were more than alarming: sixty-three men died on that day and lines of sick men were still arriving at the hospital. According to Dr. Cole's recollection of his visit to Camp Devens, one could pick out the infected men among those standing about, merely by

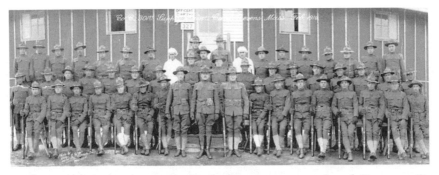

14. Captain Sylvester Benjamin Butler (front row, center) and Company C of the 301st Supply Train, 75th Division at Camp Devens, Mass., 1918.

noting the color of their faces. Many of the flu victims had displayed varying degrees of heliotrope cyanosis—a lavender hue of the face. So many soldiers had reported sick at the camp that neither the hospital facilities nor the medical staff were adequate to handle the emergency. A large proportion of the nurses, who provided the most important contribution to the care of the victims, in terms of comfort, warmth and personal hygiene, were themselves exhausted and many were also sick with influenza.[43]

Like cord-wood, the bodies were piled up at the morgue waiting to be examined. Practically all of the cadavers probed by the pathologists and medical experts showed large areas of wet, hemorrhagic consolidation in the lungs. Most of the influenza deaths were apparently the direct result of pneumonia.[44] In some cases, where death had occurred within 48 hours of onset, the lungs were filled with an enormous quantity of thin bloody fluid. This was a new and unusual observation, upon which Welch commented "This must be some new kind of infection or plague."[45]

It was a depressing time for the doctors. Welch was acknowledged to be the most stalwart of men in the face of death on a large scale, but Cole recollects that "it shocked me to find that the situation, momentarily at least, was too much even for Doctor Welch."[46]

In a little over a month's time, Camp Devens registered the statistics shown in Table 3.1:[47]

Table 3.1 Rise and Fall of the Epidemic at Camp Devens
Sept. 12–Oct. 18, 1918

	Duration Days	Cases Influenza	Cases Pneumonia	Deaths
Rise (Sept. 12-19)	8	3,283	43	16
Peak (Sept. 20-21)	2	2,722	205	43
Rapid Decline (Sept. 22-29)	8	3,141	1,495	298
Slow Decline (Sept. 30-Oct. 18)	19	571	571	310
Totals:	37	9,717	2,314	667

One out of five men at Camp Devens was ill during the autumn months. And, as Table 3.1 indicates, most of the cases occurred within a two-and-a-half-week period beginning on September 12 and ending on September 29.[48] Three-fourths of the pneumonia cases and half of the deaths occurred during that period. The doctors knew that any movement of troops to and from Devens would spread the terrible epidemic to the other camps—and, of course, already had. Welch made a call to the Surgeon General's Office in Washington, warning of what was to come, and urging that "immediate provision be made in every camp for the rapid expansion of hospital space."[49] Even with forewarning, all that could be done within the crowded camps was to prepare for the worst and wait for it to happen.

Although the nation's camps showed considerable variation in the total number of soldiers attacked, there were 306,719 cases of influenza among the American troops on this side of the ocean in the short period from September 12 to November 1, 1918. Besides the sufferers of "uncomplicated influenza," there were 48,079 cases of pneumonia, and 19,429 deaths. The statistics indicate that, as in Camp Devens, one out of five Army men had contracted the disease; of those who became ill, approximately one in six had pneumonic complications, and two-fifths of those with pneumonia died.[50] The U.S. Navy's training camps were similarly affected. After the war,

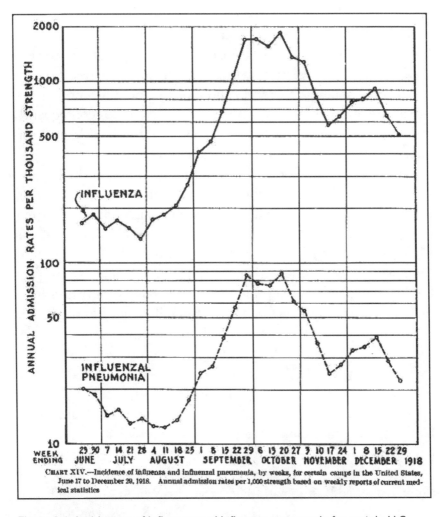

CHART XIV.—Incidence of influenza and influenzal pneumonia, by weeks, for certain camps in the United States, June 17 to December 29, 1918. Annual admission rates per 1,000 strength based on weekly reports of current medical statistics

Figure 3.1 Incidences of influenza and influenza pneumonia for certain U.S. Army Camps, June 17 - Dec. 29, 1918.

Welch was to refer to influenza as a "great shadow cast upon the medical profession."[51]

What was it like to be at one of these training centers when the pandemic began its ominous sweep? One of the nurses assigned to the Great Lakes Naval Training Center hospital, Josie Mabel

Brown, arrived there to find all the beds full in the ward and "boys that were laying on the floors and on the stretchers waiting for that boy in the bed to die."[52] The future newsman, Robert St. John, was at the Great Lakes Naval Station that September. By the time he came down with influenza, there was "no room at the inn" –not a space left in the hospital or in any of the sick bays. He was consequently assigned a cot, one of several thousand, in a drill hall. Many years later he would write: "No one ever took our temperatures and I never even saw a doctor."[53] He made his first friend in the Navy as he lay there—the man on the cot next to his. For a few days they tried to help each other remain cheerful through that dismal time. One night when the fellow in the next cot was too ill to reach for his water, St. John handed him his own canteen. The next morning his new friend was dead. An orderly pulled the blanket up over his head, and two sailors came along with a stretcher to carry him away. St. John was stunned. As for St. John himself, as quickly as he could stand on his feet, the Navy medical officers gave him two weeks' leave to go home and recuperate, hoping that his own family doctor (who happened to be Ernest Hemingway's father) would tend to his needs. As he dressed to go home, he was shocked to find that his uniform fit him like a circus tent. Only after Dr. Hemingway had examined him did he learn that he had had a severe case of pneumonia.[54]

Undergoing a similar experience was a lad who would one day become a noted Boston pathologist. Shields Warren, who graduated from Boston University in the spring of 1918, was, the following autumn, in the Artillery Corps at Camp Zachary Taylor. Flu hit the Kentucky camp in October, and struck Warren towards the end of the month. One morning he got up "feeling like hell." Somehow he managed to get as far as the parade ground, but he didn't quite make the line-up. As he put it, "when I woke up I was in the base hospital." Because of the devastating epidemic, medical care in the hospital was deplorable; the ailing men rarely saw a doctor. A young Tennessee mountaineer tended to Warren's needs from time to time, although when Warren asked him for some water, his attendant suggested a little moonshine would be more beneficial.[55]

Fortunately, Warren survived his bout with pandemic influenza. What remained stamped most vividly in his memory through the ensuing years was the picture of men dying in the wards, and the line of several hundred coffins outside the hospital every morning. As Warren convalesced at the Kentucky camp, he decided he would change his profession from zoology to medicine; surely a better way to practice medicine had to exist than what he had so recently witnessed. Then, when the Armistice came, the War Department allowed Warren and his fellow patients automatic discharges from the service. That way, if they were going to die, they would no longer be the responsibility of the U.S. Army.[56]

Yet it is unfair to suggest that the Army and its Medical Corps were uncaring or grossly negligent in their handling of the troops during the pandemic. To be in a responsible position at the camps was a grim experience, involving a feeling of utter frustration in having to stand helplessly, while watching so many young men die. At Camp Grant, Illinois, the Colonel who was its acting commandant committed suicide in mid-October 1918, probably as a result of the severe strain imposed on him by the pneumonia deaths. At the time of his death, five hundred young men had already died in the camp.[57] By October 31, there were 1,068 dead there. Of those who developed pneumonia at the camp, 45.7 percent died.[58]

Meanwhile, the Pneumonia Commission at Camp Pike, Arkansas, had expected a visit from the SGO inspection team of Colonels Russell, Welch, Vaughan, and Cole in the latter half of September. But, the Army medical chiefs never showed up at Pike because of their unexpected call to Camp Devens. Had they gone to Arkansas about September 22, they would have found the members of the Commission working ten to twelve hours a day, seeing increasing numbers of pneumonia admissions, and with no time left for themselves except to "tend to the mere necessities of existence."[59] Whereas two weeks earlier the cultures had shown that influenza bacilli were causing the pneumonias, now Type IV pneumoccoci seemed to be the culprits, the same as back at Fort Riley, Kansas. Furthermore, the white men who were involved, all new recruits, were country boys, small farmers—same as the Fort Riley negroes. The city boys seemed to be exempt, to possess some immunity to pneumococci that the country boys evidently lacked. While some members of the Commission believed the process of "herding the susceptibles" was causing the increased incidence of pneumonia, perhaps the normal mouth organisms, the Type IV pneumococci, were not the cause of the country boys' pneumonias. They probably had viral pneumonias. Moreover, that the country boys were the principal victims suggests that the city boys, or at least some of them, had had some exposure to the new virus in the spring of 1918, and consequently had built up some antibodies in their systems.[60]

At the same time the shift was occurring in the organism supposedly causing the pneumonias, influenza became epidemic on the base, "probably the same disease that has been raging in Europe," thought Blake.[61] Three of the Commission members—Small, Rivers, and Blake—had "light attacks" in the week preceding September 23. All apparently recovered without having to go to the hospital. But by September 24, a "terrific epidemic" of flu had burst loose at Camp Pike, some six to eight hundred cases in two days. There was little investigative work after that. The pathologist of the group, Major Opie, wrote Blake, "had his tail dragging on the ground" with five autopsies in one night, one after the other.[62]

During the following days, influenza seemed to run through the camp like wildfire—eight thousand cases in four days. Blake wrote: "You ought to see this hospital tonight. Every corridor and there are miles of them with a double row of cots and every ward nearly with an extra row down the middle with influenza patients and lots of barracks about the Camp turned into emergency infirmaries and the Camp closed...."[63] Then, following a breathing spell in the camp's epidemic—a false Armistice—for a few days, the fury of the

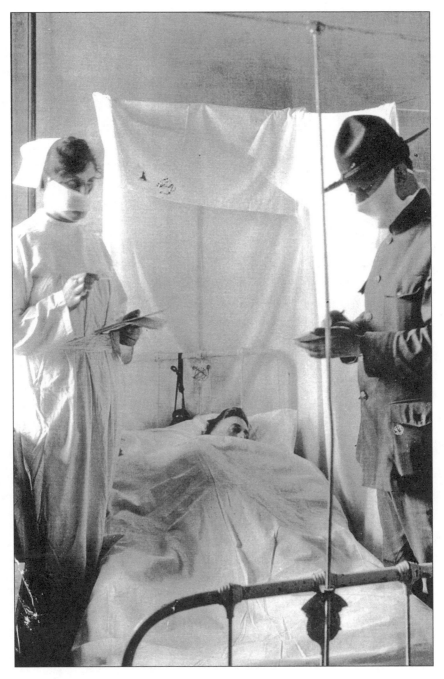

15. Soldier with influenza, Fort Porter, New York, 1918

storm let loose again. On September 30, there were two hundred pneumonia patients fighting for life in the hospital. The wards were very depressing—fifty patients in each, with not half enough nurses or corpsmen to look after them—many soldiers on cots without decent mattresses. A few days later, Blake wrote: "I am getting too tired to write about anything that is going on here. There is only death and destruction anyway."[64]

But accompanying Blake's depression was a firm belief that he and the other Commission members had an obligation to save as many lives as possible. Consequently, the five men went to see the commanding officer of the Camp Pike Hospital. The important factor was overcrowding, they told him. The incidence of pneumonia was fifty percent higher in the hospital than in the barracks. Men were crowded eighty to ninety in the hospital wards, whereas in the barracks each man had a hundred cubic feet of air space. The morgue already looked like the worst description of the London plague.[65]

The Commission members had their way. A big adjoining group of barracks became a hospital annex. Orderlies evacuated all but the measles, meningitis, surgical, and pneumonia cases from the main hospital building. Each ward was to have an absolute limit of forty patients, thirty inside and ten on the porch. Every patient would be cultured upon admission, and the streptococcus carriers would be separated from the rest. Beds were to be separated by sheets, and a strict contagion routine established. All of this meant, of course, a tremendous amount of extra work at a time when there were 4,500 patients needing care, one-third of the medical corpsmen down with influenza, and many of the professional nurses on the sick list. It took a few days to accomplish, but the reorganization did produce encouraging results. Lives undoubtedly were saved.[66]

By the middle of October conditions at Camp Pike were much improved. Whereas the deaths had been as many as thirty-five a night, there were now fewer than ten. Of the eight hundred or so pneumonia victims in the hospital, most were in the convalescent stage. Big trucks loaded with soldiers were making rounds in the evening providing jazz and close-harmony singing. The trucks had streamers on the sides with the message "Cheer up—Kill the Flu." Life was beginning to come back into the camp.[67]

The distressing conditions found in the military hospitals across the nation were also part of the scenario occurring in the civilian hospitals. As the numbers of admissions mounted day after day in the city institutions, the rosters of physicians available for duty grew smaller and smaller. At the Presbyterian Hospital in New York City, all but the youngest and oldest members of the medical staff had influenza almost simultaneously. Fortunately, only one staff member there died. The two doctors who remained well through that difficult time had to manage the entire medical service by themselves. About all they were able to do was to separate the critically ill pneumonia victims from the others, by putting them at one end of the ward. The only "treatment" attendants were able to offer the patients was to muffle them if they coughed too much. For what seemed like an eternity, each morning when the doctors made their rounds, all of the men in the critical section would be gone, all having died during the night. Finally came the mornings when first one and then a few more of the pneumonia victims were still alive. Slowly the fatalities began to lessen, and the influenza epidemic appeared to be at an end.[68]

It is worth noting that during the pandemic sick physicians often received no better treatment than the average doughboy. Captain A.R. Dochez of the Rockefeller Institute, who had been studying the bacteriology of pneumonia under Dr. Rufus Cole since 1910, and who had investigated the post-measles streptococcal pneumonias at Camp Bowie, Texas, in December 1917, found himself ordered by Surgeon General Gorgas to Camp Upton, Long Island, in September 1918 to look into the outbreak of influenzal pneumonias. Expecting to find the bronchopneumonias were the result of streptococcal infections, he found instead practically no growth on the cultures he had planted. Under the microscope no streptococci showed up at all.[69]

The morning after his puzzling laboratory findings, he began to feel ill. Thinking a little exercise would probably perk him up, he began walking over to the camp, located about a mile and a half from the hospital. However, after fifteen minutes he could go no farther, and he sat down where he was. In a little while he managed to get back to his quarters, where his thermometer revealed a temperature of 102.5 degrees—undoubtedly influenza. The camp hospital staff located a bed for him, but came round after a week to claim the space for another victim, "up and out," in other words.[70]

Captain Dochez was still so weak that he could hardly stand on his feet, much less carry the heavy bag of medical equipment which he had originally brought with him, on a three or four-mile trek to the railroad station. Ambulances were simply unavailable. Somehow he managed to coax a ride to the station from a passing Red Cross man. When he got there, the sick physician had to sit for a long while, waiting for a train that was interminably late in starting. Then, to add to his difficulties, he did not find a seat on the train when it did leave; he had to stand at one end of the car alongside his bags. By the time the train arrived in Mineola, Long Island, he had practically collapsed on the bags. But then, and happily for him, a colleague at the Rockefeller Institute boarded the train and promptly took him under his wing. Captain Dochez's destination became the Rockefeller Hospital, where he remained bedridden for a considerable period of time, followed by an additional convalescence in the country. Were it not for the rescue by his associate, it is likely that someone would have found him unconscious on the street.[71]

In the fall of 1918, flu struck so many victims without warning, at their work or on the street, that fear of disease became almost universal. Consequently, Surgeon General Blue of the Public Health Service suggested that—for their own protection—people ought to keep away from crowds. A walk to work would be healthier and safer than getting into a packed streetcar. Despite the wartime scarcity of gasoline, many automobile-owners used their vehicles to avoid contact with strangers who might give off deadly germs.[72] When Robert Frost traveled with his family to Amherst on October 4, they traveled in a neighbor's automobile. The following day Mrs. Frost wrote to Lesley: "Guess how we got here yesterday! Mr. Howes brought us down all the way in his Ford. Papa thought we would run less risk of infection than coming by train, but o, it was a tiresome trip."[73]

Mrs. Frost was highly agitated. Earlier that week when an anticipated letter from Lesley had failed to arrive at their New Hampshire home, she had been "nearly crazy for a while until papa telephoned to Mrs. Wanvig" and learned that Lesley was alright.[74] Mrs. Frost wrote that her nerves had been on edge and that her endurance had about reached the limit, on account of her worry and suspense. There was Lesley's younger sister, Irma, who had been quite sick, and was all alone among strangers. Irma had developed abscesses in her ears, and it would be several weeks before she would be able to study again. And now there was Lesley to worry about, since there seemed to be no place for her to receive proper medical care. "You must write a postal more often, dear," the mother pressed. "I must know how you are nearly every day just now when everything is as agitating."[75]

When the pandemic had begun its deadly march across New England in September, the U.S. Public Health Service had sent out telegrams to all of the nation's State Health Officers for information concerning the prevalence of influenza in their respective states. In order to help the state health offices disseminate information about the disease, Washington officials prepared a pamphlet giving the facts known about its spread and methods of prevention. Six million copies were printed, translated into many languages, and sent out for distribution. Posters that showed people using handkerchiefs were printed and circulated with the assistance of the U.S. Post Office Department and the American National Red Cross. A newspaper article was also prepared for distribution to ten thousand papers. The Public Health Service intended that the American public should know what to do if suspicious colds or influenza developed: Go To Bed At Once. Or, better yet, avoid infection in the first place.[76]

Insurance companies also circulated information about influenza to the public, via their local agents. On September 21, Dr. Lee K. Frankel, Third Vice-President of the Metropolitan Life Insurance Company, sent a telegram to five hundred company managers asking them to tell their agents to urge policyholders that they maintain good physical condition and avoid crowded places. If they were stricken, they were to go to bed and call a physician immediately. The managers were to give a copy of the telegram to each agent to be read to policyholders. Subsequent bulletins from Surgeon General Blue, Dr. Frankel informed them, would be carried in their local newspapers.[77]

But so much literature about the perils of influenza created perhaps as much fear as reassurance. A Californian was so concerned about the continual references to disease in the newspapers that he sent the following telegram to the White House:

San Diego, Calif., Sept. 26, 1918

The President:

It lies within your power to save thousands of lives by preventing all publications from printing any article mentioning epidemics or Spanish influenza. The power of suggestion for good or evil is generally acknowledged. Fear makes people susceptible. These published accounts fill the people with fear with fatal results.[78]

His plea went unheeded. In fact, the *Washington Post* began to print, usually on page one, the names, ages, and addresses of those in Washington area who had died from influenza and pneumonia the previous day, and continued the practice until the epidemic began to wane about the first of November. On Tuesday, October 8, the

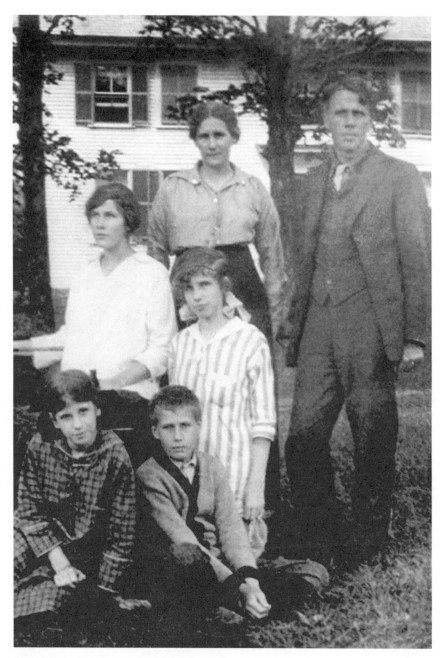

16. Robert Frost with his family, 1915

Post noted "40 Deaths Day's Toll Here" for the day before. And, a cursory glance down the column would have been enough to inform any reader that those who were dying were almost all young adults. Sixteen of the forty were aged twenty to twenty-nine, and another sixteen were between thirty and forty.[79]

Washington, D.C. did not have its first influenza related death until September 21, when John W. Close, a railway brakeman, died shortly after returning from a week's vacation in New York.[80] Until that date, Washington, D.C. residents had merely been reading the ominous reports from New England and the Middle States. First affected in the area were the military camps: on September 25 Camp Meade, Maryland reported it had an outbreak of five hundred cases of flu. The announcement prompted the District Health Department to keep a "spot map" to monitor possible troubled areas.[81]

A few days later—when the number of influenza victims had reached 1,500—Camp Meade, Maryland, the nation's largest camp with its 50,000 troops, decided to put a quarantine into effect.[82] One person who was there at the time was Henry L. Stimson. Over five hundred of the twelve to thirteen hundred men in his Thirty-Second Regiment became ill practically at once. Colonel Stimson decided to make sure that the men would receive adequate care. During the critical pandemic period, he "extemporized" his own ambulance service and, on one day alone, his emergency cars and trucks took ninety of his men to the hospital. Every day the concerned colonel went to the hospital to personally oversee the care of his men. Despite decent care, however, twenty-one died. And when all of his doctors themselves became sick, Stimson borrowed a doctor from another unit and carried on with him, some veterinarians, and dentists.[83]

Meanwhile, as the epidemic was reaching alarming proportions at Camp Meade, the American National Red Cross in Washington, D.C. decided to act upon the numerous requests for additional nurses it was receiving from New England. On September 25 the Red Cross called a meeting of various medical agencies in the D.C. area to draw up preliminary plans for affording nursing relief around the country. The U.S. Army, U.S. Navy, the U.S. Public Health Service, and American Red Cross representatives in attendance decided that the American Red Cross would supervise nursing services for the duration of the crisis. The nurses would be shifted to the geographic areas where the need seemed to be greatest.[84] The following day, Surgeon General Blue also received an appeal for extra physicians from Massachusetts. Blue did send a number of the Service's commissioned officers to the Bay State, but when calls began streaming in from other states, he knew that he had neither the men nor the money to handle the crisis.[85]

By the twenty-sixth of September, influenza was present in twenty-six states. New England had reported more than one thousand deaths within the previous ten days.[86] Many of the cities and towns in the Northeast had closed their schools, churches, and theaters, and had cancelled parades and public meetings. A considerable number of citizens in the affected areas had taken to wearing gauze masks. The general situation throughout the entire country had become so critical that the Army cancelled an order sending 142,000 men to the training camps.[87] One Red Cross report concluded, "A fear and panic of the influenza, akin to the terror of the Middle Ages regarding the Black Plague, [has] been prevalent in many parts of the country."[88] On the twenty-seventh of September, only thirteen of the military camps were still without flu.[89]

By that date, however, Congress had already stirred into action. On the twenty-first of September, Senator John W. Weeks of Massachusetts introduced a resolution appropriating one million dollars to the Public Health Service to help battle the flu. The Senate and the House had adopted the resolution the following day after only two hours' debate. When Ohio Representative Nicholas P. Longworth had revealed during the short debate that both Speaker Champ Clark and Rep. Claude Kitchin had already taken to their beds with the disease, the legislators realized that they themselves might be the next victims.[90]

The emergency medical bill (Public Resolution No. 42 – 65th Congress, and House Joint Resolution 333) was signed into law on October 1, 1918. It enabled the U.S. Public Health Service to pay for the services of the professional medical help it was recruiting across the country, and to provide that help with medical and hospital supplies, printing, clerical services, rent, and transportation costs.[91] Besides the money allocated by Congress, the American National Red Cross made an appropriation of $575,000 on October 1 to pay for the salaries and expenses of the nursing personnel it was enrolling. Later the Red Cross also offered to furnish the emergency hospital supplies that were urgently needed across the country.[92]

Three national agencies, the U.S. Public Health Service, the American Red Cross, and the Council of National Defense, coordinated the struggle to keep the pandemic under control. With the nation's Public Health Service so small, much of the organization in the cities and towns became the work of the Red Cross chapters

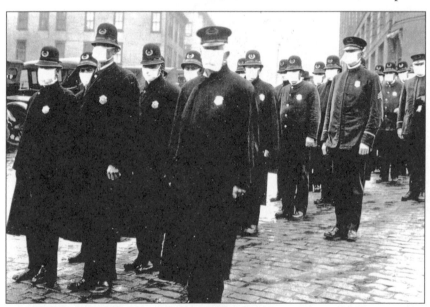

17. Policemen in Seattle wearing masks, 1918

and the local Committees of Safety and Defense. The services provided by the nursing corps of the Red Cross were particularly vital because so many of America's professionally-trained nurses had entered the military service and were unavailable for duty in their home communities. Indeed, many of the current accounts in nursing journals of the day describe how they coped during the pandemic, even though their resources were depleted by the military's needs. It was observed by Permelia Murnan Doty, Executive Secretary of the Nurses Emergency Council, reviewing the work of the Council in New York City that:

> The resources of the city would doubtless have been taxed to the utmost under ordinary conditions in an attempt to cope with the serious situation brought about by the epidemic, but at that time, because of the great shortage of doctors and nurses due to war needs, the task was one of unprecedented difficulty.[93]

Those who did yeoman service in this country during the pandemic were, in many instances, practical nurses and lay women volunteers who had taken the Red Cross course in "Home Hygiene and Care of the Sick." They now carried on under the direction of enrolled Red Cross nurses.[94] Statewide coordination of medical assistance was, in essence, a cooperative undertaking of the American Red Cross and the U.S. Public Health Service, with lay assistance from the State Councils of Defense. Meetings were held in many of the major cities in early October of 1918, to decide how best to coordinate the nursing services that were available.[95] The experiences of the nurses throughout the literature emphasize the enormity of the crisis. Mary Westphal, of the Visiting Nurse Association of Chicago explains:

> One day a nurse who started out with fifteen patients to see saw nearly fifty before night. In District 28, where the streets are

narrow and the people many, sixty-five calls were made in one day, though not of course all by one nurse. Fourteen calls in a busy season is a fair average for this small district. The Visiting Nurse repeatedly started out in the morning with a definite list of calls in her hand, but sometimes before getting out of her first case, she was surrounded by people asking her to go with them to see other patients. Physicians could not get around to all of the people needing them, it was impossible to get orders, consequently the nurse had to try to be many things to all people.[96]

The dedication of the many volunteers who worked alongside the nurses was often mentioned.

Many young women occupied during the day gave up their evenings, Saturdays and Sundays, and it was hard to turn down the enthusiastic volunteer who had already been at work all day but who insisted that she was able to sit up all night with a sick family, and work the next day.[97]

The importance of the contribution of nurses and their associates during the pandemic cannot be overstated.

As October 1918 began, the situation in Washington, D.C. grew more serious. Newspapers had reported seven flu deaths on the last day of September, and thirty new influenza victims in the district jail. To reduce the risk of contagion for federal employees who had to travel on crowded public transportation every day, various government departments implemented staggered work hours.[98] On October 2, the U.S. Treasury Department circulated new rules requiring the airing of buildings twice a day. Employees were not to spit on the floor, and were required to use handkerchiefs when coughing or sneezing.[99]

On October 3, Treasury officials received a memo reminding them that October 12 was "Liberty Day." Would they please release as many employees as possible from duty on that Saturday to let them participate in the scheduled festivities?"[100] The primary activity on that day would be to put the Fourth Liberty Loan campaign over the top, but just one day after receiving this notice, Treasury officials received another, announcing the cancellation of all outdoor meetings in the District.[101] All parades and public meetings scheduled for October 5 and 12 on behalf of the Fourth Liberty Loan would have to be cancelled. No one was more upset with the announcement than Secretary of the Treasury William G. McAdoo, whose colossal task it was to raise six billion dollars within three weeks' time.

Also on October 2, the District's Health Officer, Dr. William C. Fowler, had gone home with a bad cold, which some friends feared "might develop into influenza."[102] The District's schools and theaters were still open and the D.C. authorities were assuring the public that "there is no occasion for panic."[103] But the schools did close the following day, probably because so few parents were permitting their children to attend. At the Woodburn School in Takoma Park, Maryland only thirteen students out of an enrollment of one hundred and forty had been present the day before.[104] Following the shutdown of the schools came that of the theaters, movie houses, and public dance halls, with the warning that churches would probably follow next. Despite protests from the clergy, they, too, eventually had to shut their doors.[105]

One person who no longer cared whether the theaters were open or not was the actress, Eva Le Gallienne, who had been forced to give up her role in *Tilly of Bloomsbury* after the new play's second performance at Washington's Poli Theatre. Her illness was, of course, influenza. The upshot was that she was fired—an all-too-frequent theatrical practice at the time. However, Miss Le Gallienne was more fortunate than some of her thespian friends, for the manager paid her doctor bills and expenses for the three weeks she lay ill in a nearby Washington hotel. At the end of that time, a friend who came to take her back to her New York apartment had been thoughtful enough to have a wheelchair at the station and a drawing room on the train. He was of even more help when they arrived at her building, carrying her up the four flights of stairs to her apartment. She was still so weak that she could scarcely stand on her feet. Like so many victims, the actress had "wobbly legs." Those four flights of stairs kept her from venturing out for many weeks to come. Then, when she finally did begin to work again, she had to beg to be allowed to sit as much as possible at the rehearsals.[106]

While Miss Le Gallienne lay ill in her Washington hotel room, the District became a Sanitary Zone, with Dr. H. S. Mustard in command. Transportation facilities in the area had by now become seriously affected by the increasing numbers of ailing motormen and conductors. In order to accommodate the many sick telephone operators and female war workers, some workers' dormitories became emergency sick bays. The District banned children from the playgrounds. Following that announcement came one from the Treasury Department directing that no new war-workers could enter the area for the duration of the epidemic. On October 7, shortly after the U.S. House of Representatives announced a ten-day recess, the Chief Justice called off the Grand Jury Session for a similar period. Next, local colleges and universities called off classes and athletic contests, including the Saturday football games. Then, racing officials at nearby Laurel Track closed its gates.[107]

Like the base hospitals at the Army camps, the Washington, D.C. area hospitals proved unequal to the task before them. Thousands of victims needed institutional care. The problem was especially critical because so many residents of the area were temporary dwellers, attracted by the unusual war-related employment opportunities. Many of the young men and women who lived in boardinghouses were without family or friends to tend to their needs as they fell ill. Katherine Anne Porter was probably writing from experience in her novelette about the pandemic, *Pale Horse, Pale Rider*, when she put the following words, referring to a sick tenant, into the mouth of a boardinghouse owner: "I tell you, they must come for her *now*, or I'll put her out on the sidewalk.... I

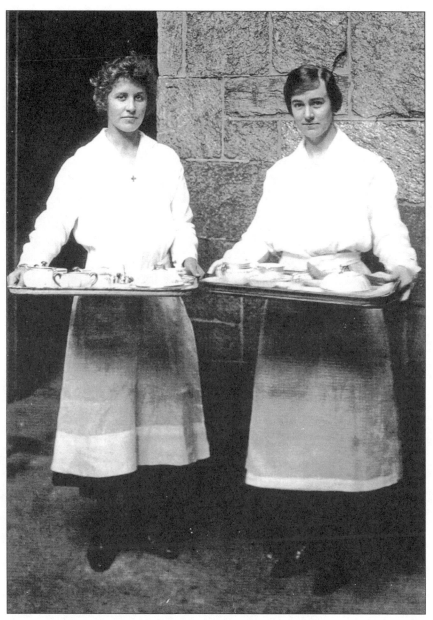

18. Two Philadelphia "society girls" volunteer during the influenza
pandemic. The city lost 12,000 during the peak weeks of September
20–November 8, 1918.

tell you, this is a plague, a plague, my God, and I've got a houseful of people to think about!"[108]

While Mrs. Woodrow Wilson was sending a rose to each female government flu victim, some of the young people in the District were dying of sheer neglect.[109] A boarder from Chelsea, Massachusetts, was dead in her room in D.C. for almost twenty-four hours before the landlord found her body. She supposedly had been "slightly ill" for several days.[110] Another Washington roomer, whose influenza had developed into pneumonia, became delirious, jumped out a third-story window, and broke his neck. He was dead a half-hour later. This unfortunate thirty-six-year-old man never had medical attention during his illness, even though other residents of the boardinghouse were aware that he was ill.[111]

Besides the construction of temporary sick bays and first-aid stations, the District issued warnings to landlords that they would be prosecuted if they failed to heat their buildings.[112] An emergency transportation system to get the sick to local hospitals and to take medical personnel to the homes of the victims soon took effect. Car owners volunteered their automobiles and themselves to keep the operation running smoothly.[113] When hospital space ran out in the District, health authorities hurriedly constructed a 500-bed unit at 19th Street and Virginia Avenue. That structure was soon filled to capacity, and twenty-five portable hospitals, similar to those used by the A.E.F., were put up on Georgia Avenue, making available another 350 beds. The War Department, which provided the nurses for the portable units, also sent fifty soldiers from Camp Humphries, Virginia to act as orderlies.[114]

Before long, soldiers at Camp Meade, Maryland were providing another service for the District of Columbia: they were making coffins to bury the dead. Like so many other large American cities, Washington ran out of caskets within a week or two after the onset of the pandemic. By October 10, the *Post* was reporting the great difficulty that undertakers were having in replenishing their mortuary supplies. For example, at Walter Reed Hospital, a score of bodies had to be kept temporarily in the morgue for want of coffins. There were now two serious public health problems—the care of the sick, and the burial of the dead.[115]

Along with banning public meetings, many of the nation's communities were now forbidding public funerals. Washington followed this course. However, some municipalities, such as New Haven, Connecticut, not only kept their schools open, but allowed public funerals, like the stately rites held for the Rev. Walter S. McElroy in the cathedral-sized St. Francis Church on October 30, during the peak of the epidemic in that city. Two hundred clergymen from all over the state took part in the long processional; 1,800 mourners were seated in the church, with fully as many more standing outside, all there to pay tribute to a popular young priest whose death from pneumonia had come the very day his military commission had arrived.[116] As his solemn funeral Mass was sung that morning, an impressive double funeral for two teaching nuns was being celebrated across the city in the Church of the Sacred Heart.[117] Meanwhile, the body of a dead woman lay in a house in nearby West Haven for seven days because the family undertaker could not obtain a casket.[118]

The coffin situation became so acute in Washington and Philadelphia that the undertakers' associations were accused of being a "coffin trust." The problem seemed to be two-fold: the short supply, and the high rates being charged by some unscrupulous believers in "free enterprise." Evidently more than a few undertakers thought that raising their funeral charges during the pandemic was only part of the natural law. When commodities were in great demand, then the prices naturally went up. As soon as signs of "profiteering" became apparent, however, the government stepped in to investigate. The survey undertaken by federal authorities revealed that a wide range of prices for funerals prevailed in the District of Columbia, with most of the burial charges ranging from one to two hundred dollars. In one instance, the exorbitant sum of three hundred fifty dollars had been levied for the casket and funeral service conducted for a young government worker. According to one federal official, "Such preying on unfortunate families in this direful time is nothing short of ghoulish in spirit and unpatriotic to the point of treason."[119]

Soon thereafter, the U.S. Department of Justice began to investigate whether a trust did, in fact, exist among the undertakers' associations or perhaps among the coffin-manufacturers. At the same time, the District's Health Officer suggested to the local undertakers that he might be forced to appoint a funeral administrator, with authority to pool the resources of the city, and to take general charge of the situation. Within a few days of these announcements, the D.C. health authorities made arrangements with a local mill and metal-working firm, whose owners promised to supply the city with at least twenty coffins a day. Finally, on October 14, Health Officer Fowler commandeered all coffins in the District, henceforth, requiring all undertakers to requisition their supplies through his office.[120]

Another aspect of the burial crisis was the serious shortage of gravediggers in the nation's cemeteries. Bodies were piling up in cemetery vaults, waiting to be interred.[121] In Connecticut various city engineering crews were put to work digging graves. Philadelphia resorted to using inmates from the Bucks County

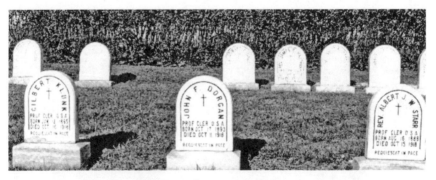

19. Graves of three seminary students in the Augustinian Community Cemetery on the campus of Villanova University. The students died of influenza within six days of each other in October 1918.

House of Correction. In many sections of the country the military undertook to help the civilian sector by sending soldiers to do the digging.[122]

In Philadelphia, death carts roamed the city. At times the city morgue had as many as ten times as many bodies as coffins.[123] One survivor remembers:

So many people died until they were instructed to ask for wooden boxes and to put the corpse, the people on the front porches. An open truck came through the neighborhoods and picked up the bodies.[124]

At "Potter's Field," a steam shovel was used to dig trenches for mass graves to bury the poor and friendless. The bodies were tagged for subsequent identification in case there was a chance that families would have an opportunity to move them later.[125] Getting a person buried was no easy accomplishment during the pandemic.

Naturally, most affected by the burial crisis were the poor. People talked not only about the "high cost of living," but also the "high cost of dying."[126] The superintendent of Washington's Central Union Mission expected that his mission's work would be greatly increased after the pandemic had subsided, for "the slender bank accounts of many families, saved by pennies and sacrifices were wiped out, and many went into debt for the burial of their dead ones."[127]

Burial supplies for the civilian sector were so scarce because the War Department continued to requisition such large quantities for its own use for the war in Europe. The pandemic created serious problems for that Department. General Peyton C. March, whose task it was to see that the A.E.F. grew in might as quickly as possible, cabled General Pershing on October 10: "If we are not stopped on account of influenza, which has passed the 200,000 mark, you will get the replacements and all shortages of divisions up to date by November 30."[128] The very week March sent that telegram, four out of every thousand men in the United States camps died of influenza and its complications. Pershing, meanwhile, was cabling for additional hospital units to be sent abroad. Finally, on October 23, March had to wire the A.E.F. chief: "Epidemic has not only quarantined nearly all camps, but has forced us to cancel or suspend nearly all draft calls....Only a few thousand replacements for November are in service...."[129] Two days later, March cabled Pershing again that every man at Fort Oglethorpe who was available for overseas duty was being sent. The personnel officer March had sent to the Fort "took all men out of organizations far down on priority to fill organizations high on priority," all, that is, who were not in the clutches of disease.[130]

Yet, if the Army personnel from Fort Oglethorpe, Georgia and other camps were healthy when they boarded the transports bound for Europe, too many of them died before the vessels docked on the other side. While the pandemic raged, a total of 789 deaths were reported to have occurred on the transports and cruisers, a number open to question. Some records suggest that only a small number, 28, were buried at sea; the rest were either interred abroad or returned for stateside services, although some of the literature of the time disagrees with this figure. One report from the Cedric, sailing from New York in October 1918, mentions 60 burials at sea on the Adriatic, a sister ship in their convoy.[131] In any case, U.S. Navy statistics showed that 8.8 percent of the troops who sailed during the autumn months became ill, and of those who had cases of influenza or pneumonia, 5.9 percent died. The Army's death rate for the voyage was 0.57 percent, meaning that one out of every two hundred men died in transport that fall.[132]

Medical officers in both the Army and the Navy urged at the height of the pandemic that the flow of troops be temporarily suspended, but the movement remained on schedule. Consequently, September through November 1918 was a grim period for the Navy. Gangplank medical inspections became the rule for those boarding transports: those efforts were at best only partially successful. During the September voyage of the *George Washington*, as many as 450 men were refused permission to board the vessel. Nevertheless, on the second day out, 550 victims of influenza reported to sick call. By the time the vessel arrived in Brest, France, there had been 131 cases of pneumonia and 77 deaths. According to one account of the voyage, 101 ailing soldiers were sent to base hospitals upon arrival, "and the remainder of the troops went ashore cheering and in fighting trim."[133]

On the other hand, the experience of the men on the U.S.S. *Leviathan*, which sailed from Hoboken on September 29, 1918 would suggest that those who disembarked on the other side were not always in "fighting trim." On that ship's voyage to France, two thousand of the approximately nine thousand soldiers in transit developed influenza, and ninety-one died before the vessel reached Brest. Those who disembarked at the French port found a storm raging, and camp a long four miles away. Without some heroic efforts on the part of Lieutenant Commander W. Chambers, of the U.S. Navy's Medical Corps, who realized that many of the men were too unwell to march that far, many more than four would have been found dead along the roadside. His naval rescue mission picked up 150 influenza and 80 pneumonia victims, and another 370 men convalescing from influenza, along the road—a total of 600 men, all of them too exhausted to continue their march to camp.[134] When the *Leviathan* cleared Brest on October 9, seven bodies were still on board, and those were buried at sea the following morning.[135]

In the midst of the pandemic, a transport convoy composed of the U.S.S. *President Grant*, *Mongolia*, *Rijndum*, *Antigone*, *Pastores*, *Wilhelmina*, and *Princess Matoika* arrived at St. Nazaire, France. During the crossing twenty-six hundred men became ill. The senior medical officer on the *President Grant* said that the conditions on board ship had reminded him of the pneumonic form of the bubonic plague. Those who died before the convoy docked numbered 246. Considering that another 204 men died later on shore, the true number of deaths for the convoy might more accurately have been put at 450. Moreover, many of the stricken men who survived the epidemic had to be shipped directly back to the States.[136] The diary of a sailor on the *Wilhelmina*, who witnessed the burial at sea of a number of those on board the *President Grant*, makes grim reading:

> *October 5 – Fifteen more bodies have just been buried from the President Grant. Fifteen were buried this morning......Such a performance as the Grant has been giving us daily is one to harden one and make one think.....I confess I was near to tears, and that there was a tightening around my throat. It was death, death in one of its worst forms, to be consigned nameless to the sea.*[137]

Other vessels arrived in Europe during the fall with fewer cases of influenza and pneumonia reported in transit, but the Battle of the Flu lay ahead. Transport No. 56—the *Olympic*—arrived at Southampton towards the end of September. The troops on board had escaped infection in the States, and only nine developed flu on the crossing. However, when the men were held at Southampton Harbor for twenty-four hours before disembarking, 383 cases of the disease developed. Many of the men were severely affected, frequently showing fevers of 105 degrees at the onset. Men on guard duty were literally dropping in their tracks. The whole shipment of troops consequently was reassigned to a rest camp on a nearby English hillside. Within a week 1,900 cases of influenza had developed, with hundreds of cases of pneumonia, resulting in 119 deaths. The medical officer who had been in charge on the crossing escaped the flu—for the time being, that is. Some weeks later on November 16, the day after his arrival at the Neufchâteau medical headquarters, he reported sick with chills and a temperature of 103.6 degrees. An ambulance quickly carried the shivering physician off to Hospital No. 18 in Bazoilles, France.[138]

Because so many of the American troops had influenza even before they reached the European ports of disembarkation, incidence of the disease among the A.E.F. was somewhat less in the autumn than among men in stateside camps. Moreover, those in the A.E.F. who were considered "seasoned" troops appeared to be less severely affected than those who arrived in late summer and fall. The explanation is probably that those who had been in Europe through the spring and summer of 1918 had the disease earlier in the year. Although there were many exceptions, most of the Army personnel who had influenza during the period from April to July escaped infection in the fall.[139] Even so, the medical chiefs in the A.E.F. were relieved when the deadly fall wave of influenza began to subside about the middle or third week of October. The number of deaths from pneumonia among the A.E.F., however, remained high for a much longer period of time.[140]

The influenza pandemic had its effect on the A.E.F. in yet another way. Although some soldiers were themselves spared an attack of the disease, or perhaps recovered without any untoward complications, all of them worried about their families back home. An A.E.F. chaplain from New York, after receiving a letter from a parishioner listing the names of those in his congregation who had died during the height of the pandemic, wrote to his wife: "Child—this pandemic! I'm glad you are fortified with faith—and a camphor bottle! I hope it has not come neigh thee, nor our Bobbie." He concluded: "Why, you at home are in the midst of a thing more insidious than war! Has it been checked by now? Oh, I hope so."[141] American soldiers in France during the last four months of 1918 were often grieved to learn of the death of a wife or brother at home. Mothers and fathers worried about their soldier sons, but those soldier sons worried about their own families in the States.

The soldiers' fears were well-founded. Although the nation's health authorities constantly reassured the public throughout the fall that there was little reason to fear influenza if one took the proper precautions, some victims of the disease died within twenty-four hours of the first symptoms of the illness. In some families, multiple deaths occurred within hours, sometimes within the same household and sometimes not. A Washington family lost twin sons within one hour of each other on October 10, Peter Haddad dying at Camp Humphries, Virginia, and Paul Haddad at Georgetown Hospital in Washington, D.C. Still a third Haddad brother, twenty-eight-year-old Michael, who operated a fruit store in the area, followed them in death eleven days later.[142]

Conditions in poverty-stricken areas of the country were particularly bad. Red Cross workers in the rural counties in Kentucky and the coal mining communities in West Virginia entered cabins to find whole families moribund with the disease, without anyone well enough to feed or nurse them. In Middlebourne, West Virginia, the pandemic wiped out the entire family of seven of Mr. and Mrs. John Linza. Following the deaths of two boys within four days, the father, mother, and two other sons died the same day. The next day the baby, the last of the family, expired. Their deaths occurred during the first week of November 1918.[143] The Red Cross reported that "people [were] starving to death, not from lack of food but because the well were panic-stricken and would not go near the sick"[144]

By November 1, however, the deadly wave of influenza had evidently waned enough along the eastern coast for authorities to terminate many of the emergency bans and regulations. Churches in Washington, D.C. opened their doors on October 31. District schools began classes the following Monday, November 4, and theaters began scheduling performances that same day.

Despite the widespread prohibition of public gatherings during October, 1918 the Fourth Liberty Loan campaign was a solid success. Washington, D.C. had cancelled its Liberty Day Parades on October 12, but some flu-bound communities put patriotism above the threat of disease. In Amherst, Massachusetts, most of the community assembled on the Common on the seventeenth to pledge an impressive $450,000. Robert Frost was a bit carried away in his enthusiasm, going home only after he had pledged to buy four one-hundred-dollar bonds. "Money!" he wrote. "You'd have thought the town was lousy with it."[145]

More of a problem for some Americans that fall was the effect of the pandemic upon the elections. Each major political party had to radically alter their campaign strategies in October because of the general ban on public meetings. Party managers had to resort to local newspaper publicity, personal letters, and house-to-house canvasses. Billboard advertising also became a popular tactic, that is, for those candidates who could afford it.[146] If anything, incumbents had the edge over their opponents in 1918: their constituents knew who they were, and what they looked like. (Considering the results of the elections, perhaps familiarity was little help to the incumbents.) In the latter part of October, New York's Democratic gubernatorial candidate, Alfred E. Smith, complained that the Republicans were using the pandemic as a means to cancel his scheduled meetings in upstate areas. The incumbent Governor of New York, Charles Whitman, had to cancel most of his own engagements besides those in Albany. It was probably just as well, since either candidate would have been disappointed with the size of the audiences they would have attracted.[147]

October 1918 ended, however, with the bans on public meetings lifted in many cities and towns in the east. People began to believe that any danger was now a thing of the past. And the war news was more positive with each passing day. The nation had survived the deadly plague, and it would soon finish up its remaining European responsibilities. Surgeon General Gorgas's successor, General M.W. Ireland, had just returned with Gorgas from the European front bringing reassurance that the health of the A.E.F. was in top shape.[148] The epidemic of influenza was therefore at an end, and those that had survived or avoided it began to assume a more cheerful outlook. At Camp Pike, Arkansas, the members of the Pneumonia Commission were happy that the quarantine had ended on October 28. The officers and men on the base were now free to come and go as they pleased, and some of them were anxiously looking forward to visits from their families.[149]

4

One War Ends

To the September and October 1918 victims of the new influenza, November promised to be a more pleasant time. One such victim had been Colonel William H. Welch who, shortly after witnessing the dismal scenes at Camp Devens in late September, had had his own "innings" with the pandemic disease. After a week abed in his Baltimore home, the bachelor Colonel decided that the sea air might promote a speedy recovery. Certainly his Johns Hopkins associates in the Maryland metropolis had become an unhealthy lot. So many of the medical center's employees became flu victims practically simultaneously that the hospital decided to close its wards to all but its own and the medical school's personnel. Before the autumn wave ended, Johns Hopkins had lost three medical students, three doctors, and three nurses to the disease.[1] Consequently, Colonel Welch was probably right in believing that the atmosphere at the well-appointed Hotel Dennis in Atlantic City, New Jersey would be more conducive to a restoration of his health. His influenza had evidently localized in his intestinal tract, a course he thought rather fortunate in that a complicating pneumonia was less likely. After a week or so at the resort, the Colonel reported back on duty at the Army Surgeon General's office in Washington on October 23, feeling fit and lucky to be among the survivors.[2]

Indeed, the entire nation, quite understandably, had fretted about its health for weeks. Late in October President Wilson received a communication from New Orleans expressing concern for his well-being: "It is such a satisfaction to know you are well, in these sick days. That is one comfort we find in the high place you so perfectly fill."[3] Flu had prevented the President, who was a regular presence at Sunday services, from attending church during October, nor had there been many guests for Sunday lunch at the White House that month.[4] Over at the Willard Hotel, Vice-President Thomas R. Marshall and his entire family had been quarantined with the flu.[5] Consequently, the President was amenable to accepting a motion picture projector when it was offered him by the popular actor, Douglas Fairbanks, who had thought the Chief Executive might enjoy a little respite from the stress of the times and the prevailing flu. Fairbanks was certain that the President could order any picture or weekly review from the local D.C. exchange, and have it delivered to the White House within an hour. Private entertainment was undoubtedly the best course for the nation's Commander-in-Chief in these worrisome days.[6]

Probably no major industry in the nation suffered such a severe economic depression during the pandemic as the entertainment field. Many states followed Pennsylvania in its order to close every saloon and place of public amusement. In some communities, even soda fountains were forced to close their doors when the owners ran out of paper cups and were unable to satisfy the strict health regulations for sterilizing dishes and glasses.[7]

However, well before the wholesale pandemic-related proscriptions went into effect, certain parts of the entertainment world had felt the pinch of wartime restrictions, particularly the drain of funds from entertainment into Liberty Bonds. People believed that they ought to sacrifice their favorite types of amusement while the nation was at war. As an example, attendance at the early games of the World Series in September of 1918 was disappointingly low, and because the ballplayers had become accustomed to playing

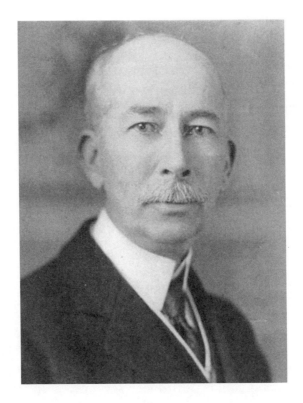

20. Colonel Edward M. House, advisor to President Wilson

before full houses, they were more than a little upset when only 19,274 fans bought tickets for the first play-off game, 13,000 fewer spectators than in the previous year. By the fifth game, the players, whose pay for the Series was based upon a percentage of the gate, were angry enough to hold up the game and threaten to call off the rest of the Series unless the owners would guarantee "full compensation." Only 24,694 people bought tickets for that contest, in the thirty thousand-capacity park of the Chicago Cubs.[8] The final Series encounter, game number six, took place in Boston on September 11, with the Sox winning 2-1. There the attendance was a mere 15,238.[9]

Although the flu had little to do with the disappointing gate receipts in the early games of the Series, it may have been a factor when the teams returned to Boston for game number six. By the eleventh of September flu was widespread in the suburbs of Boston. On the day of the final Series game, for instance, Colonel Edward M. House and his guest, Sir William Wiseman, drove from House's summer home in Magnolia, Massachusetts, to the home of the Colonel's son-in-law in Chestnut Hill, only to find him sick in bed with influenza. His illness forced the Colonel to cancel the few days' rest he had planned for himself; the two men drove off immediately to New York City, away from the flu, or so they thought.[10]

Boston and many other Massachusetts communities began to close their places of amusement, because of the pandemic, on or about September 28. Theaters, moving picture shows, dance halls, and other "unnecessary places of public assembly" were ordered closed in Boston until the sixth of October. It was estimated that the ten-day closure of the thirty-seven legitimate theaters and thirty-six moving picture houses in the Massachusetts capital would cause a loss of nearly half a million dollars to the local theater businesses, as well as a loss of tax revenue to the state government of nearly twenty thousand dollars.[11] Although several Boston stage managers said that they would pay the salaries of their house employees during the crisis, the proscriptions threw hundreds of people out of work, without a paycheck. The "Act of God" clause found in so many of the actors' contracts saved most of the managers from an awesome financial responsibility.[12]

Other eastern metropolitan areas soon emulated the Boston closings. Also cancelled were the plays and revues scheduled for many of the Liberty Theaters located in the nation's training camps. Those at Camp Devens, Upton, Jackson, Meade, Lee, and Sevier were called off early in October.[13] By mid-October theatrical performers everywhere were getting desperate. *Billboard* reported in its October 19 issue that the current theatrical depression was already the worst in stage history, and that the early ten-day bans had been renewed in most of the cities, and were still in effect. Among the states that had closed their theaters were: Massachusetts, Maine,

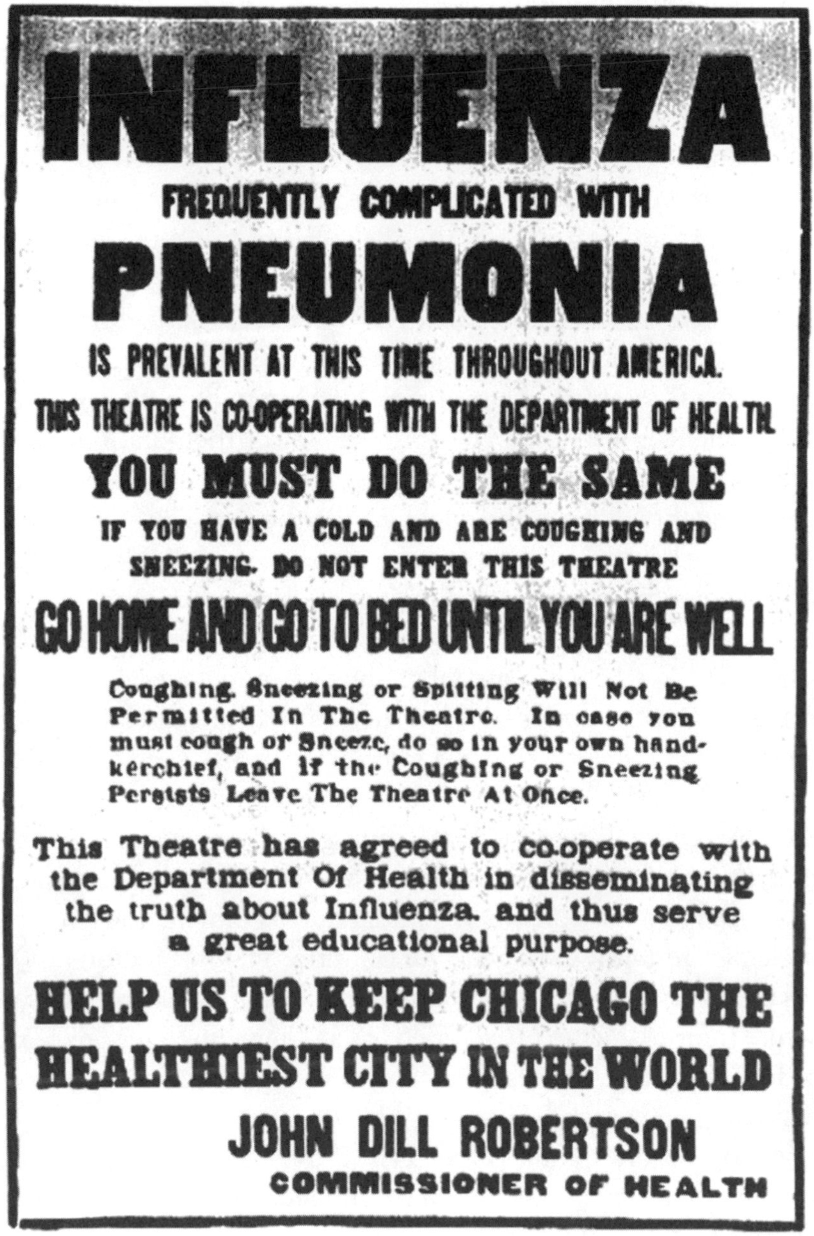

21. Poster placed in front of theaters in Chicago

New Hampshire, Ohio, Pennsylvania, Wisconsin, West Virginia, North Carolina, South Carolina, Georgia, and Florida. Theatrical performers were out of work in virtually all major cities throughout the country. Only New York City's and Chicago's theater doors were still open.[14]

Among the results of the theatrical closings were a mass invasion of those two cities by the idle performers and a tangled mess for booking agencies. *Tiger Rose*, a play running in Philadelphia when the embargo came, returned to New York City's Manhattan Opera House, where *The Wanderers* gave way with its week unfinished.[15] Unbooked theaters were a rarity in Manhattan. Nonetheless, New York audiences were disappointingly small for the duration of the pandemic. John Barrymore was starring in *Redemption*, but not even the star-quality of his name could fill the theater. The story is told that once when Barrymore became exasperated at what seemed an entire audience's continued coughing, he flung a fair-sized sea bass out into the crowd, crying: "Busy yourself with this, you damned walruses!"[16] Yet Lionel Barrymore showed more respect than his brother did for the potential seriousness of epidemic disease. During the polio and influenza epidemics occurring in 1916 and thereafter, Lionel disinfected himself in the basement of his Long Island home when he returned from the City, hoping in this way to protect his family from any deadly germs that he might have on his person.[17]

Besides temporarily crippling the legitimate theater, the pandemic seriously affected the motion picture industry. On October 14, members of the National Association of the Motion Picture Industry met in New York City and mutually agreed to cease production and distribution of new films for a four-week period, effective immediately. They hoped that they would be able to resume operations in mid-November. In the meantime, they would allow distribution of serial reels and animated newsreels in theaters not under local health embargoes. Movie houses that were still open would have to order reissues and "old favorites" for the duration of the crisis.[18]

Influenza also brought the Ringling Brothers' Circus to a halt. The far-flung quarantine forced the circus troopers to fold up their tents on their scheduled southern tour, and to move prematurely to their winter headquarters in Bridgeport, Connecticut. Fairs of every sort were similarly affected by the embargoes. The popular Danbury (Connecticut) Fair, the Virginia State Fair, the Alabama State Fair, and others due to be held in Arizona and Texas were crossed off the calendar. And "vaudeartists" across the nation often had to sit in depressing hotel rooms for weeks at a time, waiting for the bans to be lifted. Many theatrical performers were ill-prepared financially for their enforced vacations. So many actors ultimately joined the ranks of the needy that the Chicago Theater Managers Association raised a fund of $1,500 by popular subscription to help the City's idle thespians, who were also furnished meals by the local Elks while the bans remained in effect.[19]

Elsewhere, actors and moving picture house employees in Cincinnati began to seek other work situations as the weeks went by. So many of them found temporary work that the city's theater managers worried about their ability to reopen when the bans would be lifted. In Seattle the members of the Northwest Film Board of Exchanges went to work for a month in the shipyards; manager, exhibitors, and secretarial help alike were grateful to become government laborers.[20]

While the Boston theater managers chafed under their three-week hiatus, theatrical personnel in many other cities often suffered under much longer embargoes. "Willard, the Man Who Grows," finally opened his act at the *Poli Time*, Hartford, Connecticut, after an enforced vacation of six long weeks. Theaters in Canton, Ohio, were shut for seven weeks. In Terre Haute, Indiana, theater managers grew so impatient with the emergency health regulations that fourteen of them attempted to ignore the closures, were promptly arrested, and taken off to jail. After giving bond, six of the more determined men made another attempt at opening their doors. When the six were taken off to jail a second time, they decided they would leave their theaters dark, at least until their case came to court. (They won, on a technicality.)[21]

The entertainment bans lasted much longer in the west and midwest than elsewhere. Often when the theaters did reopen, annoying restrictions were still the rule, such as the wearing of protective masks, alternate seating, no smoking, and airing of the premises twice a day. Cincinnati children under sixteen were still barred from theater houses in December, and total closures were reinstated during that same month in Des Moines, Topeka, Denver, Atcheson, Wichita, Butte, Gary, and Nebraska City. Health authorities and city elders in those communities decided upon the closures and reclosures despite the growing feeling among the national medical agencies that closing theaters and wearing masks were probably ineffective means to ward off epidemics of influenza. Such advice came from the American Hospital Association as the winter progressed.[22]

As 1918 passed into history, many members of the entertainment industry were either still unemployed or working outside their normal occupations. Some unfortunates lay buried in the nation's cemeteries. It had been a truly calamitous period for the industry, providing such vivid memories that when Actors' Equity Association went out on strike in the late summer of 1919, members were determined that never again would there be a repetition of 1918's long period of financial insecurity. Equity won its case.

Another major American industry to be materially affected by the pandemic was the life insurance business. According to the historian of the American Life Convention, the influenza pandemic was to life insurance what the San Francisco earthquake had been to fire insurance. More than a few underwriters faced a severe depletion of their reserves during the pandemic; passing up the payment of dividends to shareholders became a common practice at the end of 1918. Some firms actually faced bankruptcy proceedings. Of those, the majority were eventually incorporated into the older, more highly capitalized concerns.[23]

The situation might have been worse for the industry had the government not entered the life insurance business during the war. Even before the formal entry of the United States into the war, the nation's insurance companies had considered the advantages and disadvantages of insuring military personnel. An investigation carried out within the industry in 1916 revealed that 122 of the 221 major companies had no protective clauses in their standard life insurance policies regarding military service in peace- or wartime. Those companies that already did have war clauses in 1916 charged military personnel extra premiums ranging from ten to fifty dollars per $1,000 per annum. Some of the companies simply did not insure military personnel, and a few firms refused to consider applications from any person contemplating entering the service. Still other companies would insure soldiers and sailors within the territorial United States at no extra charge, but increased the rates of individuals who left the country. As a result of the investigation, "war clauses" were almost uniformly adopted by the nation's underwriters after mid-1916. Part of the war clause recommended by the industry's investigatory board read as follows:

> During the first ten years of this policy military or naval service in time of war is a risk not assumed by the company unless the insured shall give notice thereof to the company within thirty-one days after entering on such service, and pay such extra premiums as the company may fix therefore.[24]

The new war clauses, in effect, made life insurance difficult to obtain or prohibitively expensive for the average soldier. As a result, the federal government entered the life insurance business in 1917. The new government-sponsored underwriting agency was named the "Bureau of War Risk Insurance," and operated under the auspices of Secretary McAdoo's Department of the Treasury. Members of the armed forces could purchase up to ten thousand dollars' worth of insurance from the Bureau. The industry's reaction to the government's program was mixed. Some companies were delighted that the federal government had made the decision to take the problem of war risk out of their hands, and went so far as to lend the Bureau a hand in setting up its operation; others complained that the government was interfering in private business.

Military personnel on both sides of the Atlantic quickly took advantage of the War Risk Insurance Bureau's policies. Before the war ended, the Bureau had processed approximately four and a half million applications for almost forty billion dollars worth of insurance.[25] As it turned out, this federal agency was the first insurance concern to announce the disastrous effects of the pandemic on its business. The *Washington Post* for December 5, 1918, reported that while there were no figures available yet from the private companies, the government had incurred liabilities of more than $170,000,000 in connection with the pandemic-related deaths of 20,000 American soldiers in stateside camps alone.[26]

Private insurance companies soon tabulated the financial impact of the pandemic upon their businesses. Prudential found that its death claims had tripled in October of 1918. In one day the company paid out $506,000, the most money ever handed out in a twenty-four hour period of the corporation. Each day long lines of claimants stood waiting at the company's office windows. Some of the branch offices instituted round-the-clock schedules to keep the vast reams of paper work from piling up even higher. Some funeral directors were asking for written proof that the decedent had been insured. People desperately needed money from their policies, as undertakers often required prepayment. In consequence, the insurance firms felt an obligation to settle with the claimants as quickly as possible.[27] Despite good intentions, Metropolitan Life's claim-approvers were at one time six weeks behind in their work. During the peak of the epidemic, that company received as many as five or six thousand claims a day, which was more than an average weekly load during the previous, more typical years. Metropolitan paid out approximately 68,000 death claims before the end of the year, costing the company $24,000,000 above normal for the period.[28] After the pandemic subsided, the legal reserve life insurance companies estimated they had paid out the sum of $110,000,000 in influenza and pneumonia claims during 1918.[29] Since many of the fatalities were young insurees who had been paying premiums for only a short time, many company reserves shrank rapidly.

Yet, in the long run, the pandemic was a boon to the life insurance industry. More than ever, people realized that life insurance was an essential protection for their families. Although the pandemic appeared to be catastrophic in 1918, the industry sold an unprecedented number of policies in 1919, as more than $8,000,000,000 of new business came in that year. And, within another year or two, when ninety per cent of the War Risk Insurance policies had lapsed, private companies were able to enroll many of the servicemen who had become used to the idea of paying monthly premiums for life insurance. The pandemic helped to make the average American citizen a buyer of life insurance.[30]

While the pandemic raged, a Prudential insurance agent working out of the Philadelphia office gained a reputation within the company as a man with a bright future. Doing double duty as a claims adjuster, Harry Leonard amazed his friends and fellow workers with his ability to keep up with the frantic pace. When asked how he managed to keep up the hectic schedule *and* his spirits, he replied: "I'm taking a rare old stimulant, about a pint a day. And, I'm 'way ahead on my prescription."[31]

Harry Leonard was not the only person to resort to "bottled spirits" during the pandemic. Many physicians and flu victims believed that alcoholic stimulants had medicinal value. Poor souls suffering from the chills and agues of influenza and pneumonia were often prescribed a dose of a "rare old stimulant." For the poor that stimulant was more often rum, wine, or beer than *Southern Comfort*™ or bourbon. But while Harry Leonard evidently had little trouble obtaining his bottled spirits when many of the saloons had closed, some of those at the bottom of the economic ladder found that the pandemic had cut off their normal sources of supply. Indeed, in some of the nation's communities, the pandemic afforded a "sneak preview" of Prohibition, which would come into effect in January 1920.

Many states and individual communities followed Pennsylvania in closing saloons for the duration of the pandemic. In those places, the workingman who had the habit of stopping by the corner saloon for a pint of beer at the end of the day had his routine interrupted by the health ban. Even before influenza had cut off one's "daily brew," however, alcoholic beverages had been in short supply, as the war-time Food Administration had significantly decreased the amount of grain available for production. Consequently, alcoholic stimulants were less than plentiful when the pandemic started.

Community health officials reacted to the shortage of spirits in various ways. Those physicians who disapproved of alcohol for medicinal or any other purposes were delighted to see the saloons shut down for the duration of the pandemic and the sources of supplies cut off. On the other hand, Baltimore's Health Commissioner refused to shut the saloons in his city, on the grounds that his people needed access to alcoholic beverages. A Public Health Service physician stationed in the Maryland metropolis sent the following communiqué to Surgeon General Blue:

10/11/18

Sir:

A strong and growing belief exists in the minds of the public in this city and doubtless in other cities as well where Influenza prevails, that alcoholic drinks act as a preventative of Influenza. This belief has been strengthened by the attitude of the Health Commissioner of this City, by the non-closure of saloons, giving as a reason that the people should have access thereto in order to obtain whiskey to ward off Influenza. This belief is now so strong among the laity that alcoholic drinks are being purchased and consumed in enormous quantities for the purpose of preventing Influenza. This information has come to my attention from many sources, and the use of whiskey for this purpose is being recommended by a large number of people, including some physicians.[32]

This same Baltimore Public Health Service official suggested that the time had come for a statement from the Surgeon General on the uses of alcoholic beverages, particularly on the dangers of over-imbibing. Yet the Surgeon General also received urgent requests during the fall and winter months of 1918 asking for his assistance in obtaining whiskey to be used as a medicinal stimulant. For example, Spartanburg, South Carolina's local health officers wired Blue that if he would have a shipment of whiskey sent to them from Louisville, Kentucky, the city would pay the bill and see that the whiskey was distributed by the proper authorities.[33] Surgeon General Blue wired back that his department could not act, since the requisitioning of alcohol was a matter for state, rather than national authorities. He suggested that Spartanburg should, instead, contact its State Health Officer.[34]

With the nationwide shortage of alcoholic supplies and the increased demand for them resulting from the pandemic, citizens grumbled through the fall and winter of 1918, knowing as they did that Prohibition lay ahead. In New York City, workmen appeared with "No Beer, No Work" buttons on their overalls, and residents of the Italian sector of the East Side soon displayed "No Wine, No Wedding" signs.[35] Some people seriously resented the interference in their private lives, particularly during such unhealthful times. How much of an impact this dissatisfaction had on the congressional election results on November 5 cannot be determined.

Nor can one estimate the number of voters who stayed away from the polls because of the pandemic. Twenty-five percent fewer people voted in 1918 than in the 1916 presidential election, but along with the normal decrease in the number of voters seen in off-year elections, wartime conditions, especially the lack of a regular procedure to provide for soldier voting, certainly contributed to the decline.[36] With soldiers in the camps and overseas, and war-workers employed in munitions' plants and shipyards far from their homes, a significant decrease was to be expected. Those who were sick in bed or confined to their homes, however, obviously did not vote either.

Included in the group of non-voters on November 5, at any rate, were two prominent Democrats. One was Secretary of the Treasury McAdoo, whose ten-day siege of influenza kept him from making the trip from Washington to his New York polling station.[37] And, the Secretary's father-in-law, President Wilson, also elected to remain in Washington that day instead of riding to Princeton, New Jersey, to vote for fellow Democrats.

The President's decision to remain in the White House on the fifth of November no doubt reflected the critical nature of his peace negotiations with Germany, rather than any reluctance on his part to mingle with potential disease carriers in Princeton. Before the election week came to an end, a "false Armistice" sent Americans into the streets, singing and dancing with joy. Two days after the election Thomas L. Sidlo, a former law-partner of Secretary of War Baker, sat in his Cleveland, Ohio office, dictating a letter to Baker assuring him that he and his family and friends were now on the road to recovery from their bouts with the flu. Sidlo had just finished the second paragraph, informing Baker that "Hazel is improving rapidly...Win recovered from her attack several days ago...and Joe is about through with his trouble, so that our casualty lists are looking better all the time."[38] At that point the office secretary walked in carrying under her arm an extra edition of the *Free Press*, with its headlines announcing Germany's capitulation to the terms of the Armistice. Sidlo wrote: "These are wonderful days in our history, and it must be splendid to be where one can see the sun of our triumph and glory coming up over the horizon."[39]

The Cleveland newspaper, like so many others across the nation, had picked up the premature announcement that had been wired to the States by a few overzealous newsmen on the Western Front. Nevertheless, the release merely reflected how rapidly the war was drawing to a close. By November 1 the war was, in effect, over; both sides knew it. Baker's friends in Cleveland were probably more worried about their health as November began than the optimistic report Sidlo sent to Baker would suggest. Sidlo was fortunate in that he had managed to secure the services of a student nurse to look after his wife when she had fallen desperately ill, but only by paying the novice angel of mercy a handsome forty-five dollars a week.[40] The truth was that although the East Coast seemed to be just about over the epidemic at the beginning of November, parts of the country were still in the clutches of the disease.

Sidlo's former law-partner, Secretary of War Baker, while not ill as November began, nevertheless had had his sleep interrupted by the ravages of the disease. Baker, who had made a hurried trip to Europe earlier in the fall, had been unable to call upon or talk with another old Cleveland friend, Brand Whitlock, then serving at the United States Legation in Le Havre, France. On November 2, shortly after his return home, Baker wrote to Whitlock to inform him that Whitlock's former secretary, Bernard Daley, had died at the emergency hospital in Washington. Evidently Daley had told the medical personnel at the hospital that Baker was the "nearest kin or closest friend" he had in the area, for the War Department chief had been summoned to his bedside. Baker promptly responded to the call, and promised the critically ill Daley he would return the following day. In the middle of the night, however, the hospital called Baker to inform him that Daley was stubbornly refusing to take the remedies prescribed for him: would Baker come down and try to talk some sense into the patient? However, Daley was dead of pneumonia by the time Baker got there.

The War Department head wrote to Whitlock: "I learned at the hospital that they had tried to get him to take some whiskey as a stimulant, but that he had obstinately (and I am afraid, profanely) refused."[41] Once a teetotaler, always a teetotaler, or at least so it was with the unfortunate Daley. Baker also added that Daley had been working until only three days before his death.

Despite having to relate such unwelcome news to Whitlock, Baker wrote that he was cheered by the shifting scenes in the great drama happening about them. He hoped that the new act of world events so soon to begin would be one of lasting peace. Baker added that he was an obstinate optimist: "I do believe the world is growing better—I know the United States is and that there is more idealism per capita among us now than there ever was before in our history, and so far as I know, the history of other people—more than there had been anywhere at any time."[42]

Baker's optimism as November got under way was shared by the ailing Harvey Cushing: "The news astonishes. Old world dynasties are tottering...."[43] Curiously enough, a rumor of Woodrow Wilson's assassination was making the rounds in the wards at Cushing's hospital on the very day that American newspapers were prematurely announcing the end of hostilities. Much to the doctor's relief, the unsettling report proved baseless.[44] During those last days of the war, Cushing and some of his fellow neurosurgeons serving in American hospitals in France found themselves thinking of the future. Perhaps it would be possible to organize a National Institute of Neurology upon their return to the States? Such a center would attract the best practitioners in the field, and it might someday become the model neurological institution in the country. Cushing and his associates thought the major problem would be in financing such a venture. Some of the medical men suspected it ought to be done without getting the government involved. As Cushing put it, if Congress had any brains it didn't use them—"a Congressman is nothing but a heart and a pants' pocket—just sentiment and cash, in other words."[45] For many American physicians serving in Europe, the closing days of the war were a time for grandiose dreams, that is, if they had the time to think of anything but the war and influenza casualties.

The Great War finally came to an end at the eleventh hour on the eleventh day of the eleventh month of 1918, although the signing of the Armistice had already occurred early that morning. Within a few minutes of the pre-dawn formalities, fifteen minutes to be exact, President Wilson's special envoy to the Supreme War Council, Colonel E.M. House, had been awakened in his Paris residence to be given the "glad tidings." Colonel House recorded in his diary for November 11 that he had been the "first" person notified after the signing, even before the President had received the news.[46]

But the Colonel was not the man of the hour; that man was his Chief Executive, Woodrow Wilson. The great hero on November 11, 1918 was the American President. It was truly the apex of his career. Throughout the Western world, people blessed him and revered him. Even Wilson-haters, for the moment, considered him a "super politician—and *pro tanto* a great genius...."[47] Robert Frost thought Wilson to be representative of the current sentiment in the world of those who wished to steer clear of radical ideas. As for Frost, he himself was "out to see a world full of small-fry democracies even if we have to fill them two or even three deep in some places."[48]

When Frost wrote those words to his friend, Louis Untermeyer, on October 28, the two men had been writing back and forth, somewhat in jest, about the states of their health. Untermeyer, sick in bed with influenza, had written Frost suggesting that the poet get busy on a suitable obituary in preparation for Untermeyer's fancied demise on December 17. Frost wrote back for further details about the diagnosis of his friend's disease: "Too long for influenza it seems too short for most of the critics I have heard of or for due process of law."[49]

Frost could still write lightly about the pandemic disease. Before the winter ended, however, he was to change his opinion of the prevailing illness. He was sick in bed twice during the fall, the second time very ill indeed with influenza. But, as the Armistice neared, Frost was in good spirits, impatiently waiting for all "throwns" to be "throne" down.[50]

When the "throwns" did come tumbling down that autumn, and the Germans capitulated early that November morn, Allies everywhere were in joyous spirits. Red Cross associate, Mrs. J. Borden Harriman, then in Paris, later wrote: "We were mad, that 11th of November."[51] In the words of Wordsworth, "But to be young was very heaven."[52]

There were, however, some exceptions. Another American still on French soil that morning, the aforementioned Massachusetts General Hospital nurse serving in the British hospital, who had had two attacks of influenza earlier in the year, was back in the hospital again, this time quarantined with diphtheria and trench fever. As eleven o'clock neared on November 11, she penned the following thoughts into her diary:

> In ten minutes the war will be over. Hostilities are to cease at eleven o'clock …. It's incredible that one can measure peace in actual units of time. I lay awake all last night thinking.
>
> What are we to do now? How can we go home to civilian life, to the never ending, never varying routine?
>
> There go the bells! And the drums! And the sirens! And the bagpipes! And cheering that swells louder and louder! The war is over—and I never felt so sick in my life. Everything is over.
>
> But it shan't be! I _won't_ stop living![53]

Fortunately she lived to enjoy better days. By the first of December she was well enough to leave the hospital for a period of convalescence in the south of France. When Christmas came she was back with her unit, and—before another month had passed—was homeward bound across the Atlantic. The New England nurse, incidentally, had escaped the deadly wave of influenza when it had swept through her hospital wards in October. At that time only the recently arrived Army units had "died like flies." Those like herself who were veterans were generally not very sick if and when the disease struck them.[54] "Seasoning," whatever it really constituted, did indeed seem to make a difference.

In the United States, the news of the Armistice brought people out into the streets, even where influenza-related bans were still in effect. Impromptu victory parades were very much in evidence and folks of all ages not only sang and danced, but they drank too much and they kissed numerous strangers. In the cities the raucous activities caused more than a few participants to end up in the local hospital emergency rooms. For medical personnel who were on duty that day, it was an unforgettable experience. Dr. Loyal Davis was serving an internship at a Chicago hospital where examining rooms were filled with celebrants throughout the day. After their cuts and bruises had been attended to, they were either sent home or to the city jail. All this was on top of the ravages of the still-widespread pandemic. According to Dr. Davis: "For twenty-four hours all the interns were involved in a confusion of alcohol, scalp wounds, blood, harsh dry coughs, gasping breaths, death, and squalling babies being delivered from mothers dying from influenza."[55] The young interns, who had already been sobered by the news that four of the hospital's former interns had died in military camps, did little celebrating themselves.[56] Medical people had to battle the flu *and* the drunks on that November day, and unfortunately, only one war had ended.

In small towns throughout the nation the day's festivities were often less boisterous, yet hardly less emotional. In New Hampshire, novelist Frances Parkinson Keyes, whose husband was Governor of the State and had been elected to the U.S. Senate on November 5, responded affirmatively to a call within minutes of the news of the Armistice that she participate in a parade in the village of Newbury. When she arrived, perhaps an hour or two later on a perfectly marvelous crisp autumn day, an impressive crowd had already gathered in the center of the village. As the townsfolk lined up alongside the Common, a makeshift band of local musicians put themselves in the lead. Passing by the monument to the town's Revolutionary War hero, General Jacob Bayley, paraders stopped to offer a salute. After circling the Common, they marched on to the local cemetery where they offered memorials at the graves of heroes of other wars. Eventually the group marched back to the village, singing all of the popular war tunes as they went along. Finally, "without prearrangement," they ended the parade with "Onward Christian Soldiers." A deeply emotional rendition of the hymn sounded aloft in the lakeside community that day.[57]

Some years later, the author recalled that she had been glad to have that parade to look back upon as 1918 progressed, for the weeks that followed were, in many ways, very grim indeed. Influenza soon returned and ran rampant across the state. New Hampshire's initial autumn epidemic had run from mid-September to mid-October, and as it had abated, schools and churches opened up again, and the epidemic became only a memory. But following upon the heels of the Armistice festivities, a second wave of illness seemed to take hold. Families who had escaped influenza in September and October now fell ill. In the Keyes family, Henry, Jr., came down with the disease during his Thanksgiving holiday from Milton Academy while visiting his grandmother at Andover, Massachusetts. Then, one after another, son Peter, husband Harry, and the writer herself came down with the flu, to be followed by son John when he came home for his Christmas break.[58]

So great was the demand in New Hampshire that, despite a houseful of sick people, a trained nurse was simply unavailable to the Governor's household as well. The Governor and Mrs. Keyes did have one domestic servant to bring up trays of nourishing food to their bedside, and to tend to the special needs of the children. Then, as the days passed, the out-going Governor's attack of influenza went into his lungs, and the diagnosis changed to pneumonia. But, little by little, the family regained their strength, getting up out of bed first for fifteen minutes, then for a half-hour, and finally for hours at a time. The Governor's recovery was prolonged enough, however, that he was unable to deliver his farewell speech. Thus, as the year 1918 ended, influenza was still about in New Hampshire.[59]

Another family who believed when November came that they had escaped the pandemic were the Frederic C. Walcotts, then living within commuting distance of Washington, D.C. Walcott was Herbert Hoover's assistant in the United States Food Administration. Beginning about Thanksgiving the disease took hold in the family. By the time 1919 had begun, Walcott was reporting to his brother that the family Christmas had been pretty well broken up by the flu. He was nonetheless thankful that the seven Walcotts who had been sick within a month had apparently all recovered without complications.[60]

Still others, like Robert Frost, seemed to have second attacks of the disease as the winter came on, the second one usually more severe. Perhaps the victims actually had bacterial complications, or relapses, or colds. Or possibly the first attacks had not been influenza. In any case, the parents of Thomas M. Carothers, Jr., a candidate for a U.S. Naval commission at the Great Lakes training center, believed their son was having a second attack. In early October the young man had a ten-day bout of influenza while he was aboard the *J. S. Ashley* on the Lakes and had apparently completely recovered. Then, on the first of November, the Navy transferred him to Chicago's Municipal Pier for additional instruction and training with his class. There, working and sleeping in unheated quarters, Tom and some of the other men contracted "influenza in its most violent form." They were desperately ill at the end of November. As he began his second period of convalescence, the Navy decided to give the young man a three-week leave of absence so that he might recover at home. He was placed on the train for New York one Thursday evening, and when his family met him the following afternoon, they were shocked to find him so ill and emaciated that he was unable to walk without assistance. His family thereupon took it upon themselves to ask the U.S. Navy to give their ailing son an honorable discharge, to be effective immediately.[61]

The problem of adequate convalescent care for military personnel worried many American parents that fall. Both rich and poor made gestures to the military medical authorities, offering to house some of the young men as they fought to regain their health. A Pennsylvania mother, whose oldest son had suffered a severe case of influenza despite having received every luxury and care, became extremely anxious for the lives of other mothers' sons who were far from home and perhaps in need of good nursing care. She wrote to Secretary of the Navy, Josephus Daniels, and offered to have a large country club near Philadelphia opened up as a convalescent home. The two-hundred-bed club, of which her husband was the President, had "wide porches, large amusement rooms, and a baseball field." It had closed for the season, but she would see to it that the club was reopened, financed, and run by the local chapter of the Red Cross Navy Auxiliary that she chaired. If the Navy would give some of the sick men two weeks' leave, she and her fellow members of the auxiliary would see to their proper recuperation.[62] The pandemic may have induced panic, but it also brought out the best in some citizens.

The U.S. Navy's Medical Department, which politely refused such offers, also heard from John W. Cavanagh of New York City. In the latter half of October 1918 he wrote to the Navy and offered to install in his home four double beds "for our sick boys." Mr. Cavanagh asserted that he could provide "warm beds, warm rooms, food, medicine and care without charge," as well as the services of a good nurse. He added: "I hope the rich people in this city will use their homes as I am doing. I am a poor man with eight in my family but will make every sacrifice to help our sick soldiers and sailors."[63] The kindly Mr. Cavanagh evidently had no fear that in the process he might become a victim himself.

How different was the attitude of health authorities in West Point, Mississippi, who advised absolute quarantine of every influenza patient. They contended that the healthy should stay away from the sick, and vice-versa. If Mississippi citizens ignored the present danger, they were warned, they might as a result of their "defiance of the silent foe take a trip to heaven, or some other place."[64]

In Quitman, Georgia, every person who traveled on a train was considered to be a potential harborer of the "silent foe." As a result, those who came into the city by rail were required to wear masks for four days. So, too, were new guests at the city's hotels, lodging houses, and boarding houses. In addition, any person who was fortunate enough to recover from the disease was required to don a mask for his first week back in public.[65]

Quitman's emergency pandemic-related rules and regulations, numbering twenty-seven, went into effect on December 13, 1918.[66] Georgia communities, like so many others in the Southern states, found that the pandemic grew more serious as the winter wore on. Public health officials in Montgomery, Alabama, were upset by the releases purporting to come from Washington carried in local newspapers to the effect that the danger was over. Surgeon General Blue was quoted as having said: "The country need not fear that the influenza epidemic will return. It has come and gone for good." Since the Alabama city was in the midst of a grave epidemic on December 11, the city's health officials wrote to Blue for help in remedying the local situation.[67]

Such appeals for help prompted the Surgeon General to issue a new bulletin warning the nation that influenza was still widespread. To reinforce the U.S. Public Health Service bulletin, the Council of National Defense sent out telegrams and follow-up letters to the State Councils of Defense recommending that those organizations get behind public health authorities. Community Councils were also urged to help organize in the fight against disease.[68]

Not only was influenza widely prevalent in the nation's cities and towns, but it had started up again, in what threatened to be epidemic proportions, in the military cantonments. At Camp Pike, Arkansas, the Pneumonia Commission in the period following the

Armistice had looked forward to finishing up some experiments and perhaps getting discharged from the service before Christmas.[69] On November 18 the laboratory workers had one final series of tests to run on a newly-received batch of fourteen monkeys. What they hoped to do was reproduce influenza in the animals. On the twenty-first they tagged the monkeys, took their temperatures, and made throat cultures, with the expectation that this information would provide a baseline for their experiments. A couple of the monkeys who were particularly large and vicious became "Kaiser Bill" and "von Hurdy." The temperature-taking would continue for three days, after which the doctors would spray the monkeys full of influenza bacilli. If the flu could be reproduced, then the experimenters planned to try to give the monkeys pneumonia on top of their flu.[70]

After the monkeys were sprayed with the influenza bacilli, nothing seemed to happen for a few days. Then, however, the animals became less important than what was happening in the camp. On November 28 a secondary wave of influenza began to send recruits into the hospital again. The pneumonia investigators were afraid their plans to leave Pike were about to be "knocked into a cocked hat" when they received orders to start checking out the victims of the new epidemic.[71] But the outbreak turned out to be of minor proportions—only ten to fifteen cases a day. On December 11, Captain Blake would write that the epidemic had not amounted to much: "Of course, it is quite different now from the height of the epidemic, because the wards are not overcrowded and because the influenza in general is much milder. There is however a greatly increased percentage of streptococcus carriers...."[72] Nevertheless, there were eight hundred pneumonia patients in the base hospital—hardly a trifling matter. Officials at Camp Pike decided to quarantine the post again.

As for the Commission members, their days at Camp Pike would soon end. On the fifteenth of December orders arrived for them to report to the Commandant of the Army Medical School in Washington, D.C. on December 29. By the middle of December, however, the monkey experiments had become rather interesting. The laboratory scientists had not only been able to isolate the influenza bacillus from the throat of a very sick, cyanotic animal, but had also been able to produce a Type III pneumococcal pneumonia in a few of the animals. While some of the investigators apparently were excited with the results, Blake admitted that the experimenters had not as yet been entirely successful in producing the pathological picture of influenzal pneumonia. This meant they did not have sufficient proof to stand the test of the most rigid critics.[73]

In fact, influenza research was ongoing in many centers simultaneously at the end of 1918, but such was the prevailing confusion about the cause of influenza that there was significant disagreement about the type of bacteria associated with the disease. Eight different bacteria had already been designated as the etiologic agent in influenza, most commonly B. influenzae, pneumococci and hemolytic streptococci.[74] Despite the obvious lethality of the causative agent, experiments with human volunteers were set up by a number of investigators with the aim of identifying it.[75] The volunteers were servicemen at the Naval Training Stations in Boston and San Francisco, who had been convicted of various offenses during their time in the Navy. They were offered a pardon (if they survived) in exchange for participation—such inducements may not have been considered an ethical issue in 1918. However, in spite of the best efforts of the investigators, such early human experiments yielded no satisfactory answers in regards to the identity of the influenza pathogen.

In the District of Columbia, despite the Washington Post's optimistic post-Armistice report that "one may now cough or sneeze without causing chills to run up and down the spine of chance neighbors," December brought an increase in the number of influenza cases reported to the District's health authorities. Consequently, renewed precautions were advised. By the middle of the month, when there were many absentees in the District schools, authorities considered closing them again. Washington did not do so, but many other sections of the country did. In parts of Ohio the disease was almost as prevalent as eight weeks earlier, and renewed closings of every kind became the rule. The situation in Michigan in mid-December was the worst since the onset of the pandemic. In addition, the U.S. Public Health Service now reported that it had practically used up the emergency federal appropriations. Should the disease reassume epidemic proportions across the nation, the agency would have to ask for additional funds.[76]

As the situation deteriorated in Washington, local health authorities appealed to Congress for an additional $50,000 for the District. In the meantime, an emergency flu hospital had to be opened up for the area's latest victims: the U.S. Housing Corporation provided the emergency structure. As December ended, epidemic conditions were again present in the capital, blamed now, however, on the bad weather. At the same time, Washington area residents learned some grim statistics: influenza had killed one out of every two hundred of the District's population. One of every sixteen victims of the disease had died.[77]

As 1918 drew to a close, the American people also began to get a more accurate picture of the course of the disease among the American Army in Europe. Wartime censorship came to an abrupt end with the signing of the Armistice. According to statistics released to the *New York Times* on the day following the Armistice (before the receipt of uncensored reports), 4,984 of the A.E.F. had died of disease by November 11.[78] Yet on Sunday, December 1, the *Times* called into serious question the earlier figures by reporting that 16,904 had died of disease through and including, November 26. Congress now demanded to know why the casualty lists reported thus far had not accurately reflected the true numbers of Americans killed, wounded, or otherwise incapacitated. Secretary Baker was summoned back into the witness stand to be queried about the apparent delay in reporting casualties.[79]

The influenza pandemic in the fall and winter months of 1918 undoubtedly made the gathering of such statistics increasingly more difficult for General Pershing's aides. Through November troops were still arriving at the European ports, some falling sick or dying on the way. One eleventh-hour victim was the noted author, John Dos Passos. Although he had done a stint as a volunteer ambulance driver earlier in the war, he had returned to the States, as noted previously, in August of 1918. Within a month he had convinced the Army to let him enlist, despite the notoriety he had earned in the Ambulance Corps. At the end of September he was at Camp Crane in Allentown, Pennsylvania, quarantined behind "three strands of barbed wire," washing a "million windows," and sweeping the dust off the barrack floor. The quarantine hampered his style—and his writing: "God! How can one write in captivity in quarantine?" What Dos Passos did to while away the time was to dream up a play about *Death*. In the first act *Death* was a "lousy little man rather like a doctor, with a black bag." In the next act he made *Death* a garbage man.[80]

In any event, the impatient, would-be hero described himself on October 20 as being as "bored as a polar bear in a cage."[81] But by November 1 he was at Camp Merritt, New Jersey, the first stop on the journey to France. Before he landed at Brest, he found time to record in his diary that the voyage had been more eventful that he had anticipated:

After four days of miscellaneous and most grievous disease, I feel well enough to scribble notes again. I think I've had symptoms of all known diseases: pneumonia, T.B., diphtheria, diarrhea, dyspepsia, sore throat, whooping cough, scarlet fever and beri-beri, whatever that is.[82]

Soldiers coming and going—November and December 1918 saw the first of the two million men in the A.E.F. embark for home.

On December 16, the largest of the transports, the *Leviathan*, landed at Hoboken, New Jersey carrying eight thousand American troops. The harbor was in a wild tumult as New York came out to greet the returning heroes. However, on the voyage home from Brest, four sailors and one soldier had died and the ship's surgeon reported that 150 cases of influenza had erupted. Considering the ten thousand passengers, it was a reasonable number, unless, of course, one's son happened to be among the five fatalities. But the crossing became a memorable event for many of the young men on the transport. Among the passengers was the Detroit Tigers' amazing Triple Crown winner, Captain Ty Cobb. Before he left the ship, Cobb invited his fellow voyagers to attend "some big game" in which he would be on the field. He gave them a password that would get them past the gatekeepers. They were to tell the ticket-takers they had been "on the *Leviathan* when Ty Cobb tried to make a speech during a minstrel show at sea." Oh, it was good to be home again.[83]

Despite the gala celebrations held upon the arrival of the troopships, citizens of the nation's largest city had been sobered by some pandemic-related social problems peculiar to its size. On November 8, New York City Health Commissioner, Royal S. Copeland, announced that approximately 31,000 children had already been made half or full orphans by the Spanish influenza. In 7,200 families either one or both parents had died. About 700 of those families, affecting some 2,000 children, needed financial help from the city.[84]

For those children who had lost both parents, many individuals and institutions came forward to offer temporary or permanent assistance. Some of the children needed help only until their relatives could offer proper guardianship. For others, more than fifty persons had already offered to adopt flu orphans, especially those between the ages of one and three. Also, the Hebrew National Orphan House, at 52 St. Mark's Place, announced it would take seventy-five to one hundred orphans, and the Hebrew Kindergarten and Day Nursery at 30 Montgomery St. opened a special ward for the children of mothers dead or ill of influenza.[85] A visual reminder of the ravages of the pandemic, in the form of a photo showing about twenty-five two or three-year-olds, was offered to the readers of the *Times* on Sunday, December 15. The caption read: "Living 'Christmas Dolls' Sent Last Week from New York to be Distributed Among Childless Homes in the Middle and Far West." Many of these "little waifs," the legend read, were made homeless by the loss of both father and mother in the influenza epidemic in New York.[86]

Pandemic-related poverty cases also overwhelmed the city's social agencies that Christmas season. Among the *New York Times* "One Hundred Neediest Cases" were many families who had been victimized by the pandemic. The number of destitute residents rose so high that, for the third year in a row, the *Times* published a second Hundred Needy Cases. Included among the impoverished were the following:

Case #95: "Family Stricken by Influenza"

John M., a hard-working young man, his young wife and their baby all had severe attacks of influenza. The young husband, who was run down by overwork when the attack came, developed pneumonia and is still in a hospital. His wife cannot work and the weeks of sickness have swept away their small savings. They need only a little help to give them a new start. $100 is asked.
(Reported by Charity Organization Association)

....

Case #69: "Mother, with Five Children, Ill"

Walter D., an excellent mechanic, cared well for his wife and five children, until pneumonia following influenza took his life. The next week Mrs. D. and two of the children were taken with the same disease. The death and the period of sickness used up their savings. The mother, still ill, faces the problem of caring for her five children of 7, 5, 3, and 2 years and a tiny baby. She has nothing at all now. She is eager to work, but $200 is needed to help her through the coming year. (Reported by Brooklyn Bureau of Charities)

....

Case #59: "Father a Victim of Influenza"

Influenza carried off Albert E., a conscientious worker and a good father. This occurred when his wife, whose latest child was less than a month old, lay ill with pneumonia. There are six other children in the family. The eldest, young Albert, will go to work in the Spring. The mother is barely convalescent now, and the plight of the family is desperate. They need $630 to see them through the period of trouble. (Reported by Association for Improving the Condition of the Poor)

....

Case #11: "Influenza Impoverishes a Family"

Timothy McG. idolized Bridget and Mary, his two little daughters. When they got influenza he worked day and night to get extra money for special care and food for them. By the time they had pulled through, he was tired out and ill. Three days later he died of the same disease. "He sacrificed his life for his children," the doctor told the charity worker who visited the family. Worn out by her efforts during this period of sickness, the mother is in the hospital. They have no money. $640 is needed to help them all to get well and to get started again. (Reported by Charity Organization Society)

....

Case #36: "Two Dead of Influenza"

The father died 6 weeks ago when he had to undergo an operation for appendicitis immediately after getting over influenza. It left the mother to take care of five children, the eldest 9 years, the youngest a child in arms. There was another little boy, 3 years old, who died of influenza. Stunned by these two deaths, the mother is in no condition at present to face the future. She is, however, an excellent mother, a capable housekeeper, a woman whose name is worth protecting. A little help will give her a new start. Two hundred dollars is needed. (Reported by Brooklyn Bureau of Charities) [87]

....

The social wreckage, as described in these cases in New York City reflected what took place on a lesser scale elsewhere. For example, the New England Division Headquarters of the American Red Cross in Boston received a report from its chapter in Berlin, New Hampshire that twenty-four children in that small community had been orphaned during the first month of the autumn wave of the disease.[88] In another small town in Massachusetts, there were sixteen motherless children living on one street.[89] Women in the last stages of pregnancy had evidently been particularly vulnerable. According to Dr. E. O. Jordan, the effects of influenza on pregnancy seemed to be more serious than any other known infection. Many women in 1918-19 had their pregnancies interrupted. Some died even as live babies were taken from their wombs; others delivered dead fetuses. In addition, not only were there fewer live births within the Registration Area of the United States in November and December of 1918, but fewer babies were conceived during October of 1918 than during the same month in 1917 and 1919. Interestingly enough, a similar lowering of the birth rate had been noted nine months after the height of the 1890 pandemic.[90] Spanish flu was no minor disease, certainly not one to be considered simply as "a three-day malady."

As 1918 ended, influenza was still taking its toll around the nation, having lost only its explosive character. Fear was still abroad in the land, particularly among those who had thus far escaped the disease. The question that still haunted many of them was: would they be visited by the "silent foe"? And, if so, would they be that "one out of sixteen"?

5

The "Paris Cold"

During the fall of 1918, many French Catholics circulated the theory that God had sent the influenza pandemic to restore the balance between the sexes.[1] Perhaps it seemed that way in towns where large numbers of young men had gone off to war and, as a consequence, women constituted a disproportionate share of the local influenza casualties. But the disease affected men of all ages. Robert Frost was one male victim who showed more respect for influenza as 1919 began:

> Here it is as late as this (1919 A.D.) and I don't know whether or not I'm strong enough to write a letter yet. The only way I can tell that I haven't died and gone to heaven is by the fact that everything is just the same as it was on earth...I was sick enough to die and no doubt I deserved to die.[2]

The New England poet's illness, rumored to be tubercular, was diagnosed as the flu. His first sickness in the fall of 1918 seemed to be only a minor inconvenience, and perhaps may indeed, have been a common cold rather than the flu. On the other hand, if it were the flu, he may have suffered a relapse during his convalescence, perhaps the result of a complicating pneumonia. It seems likely that Frost had serious lung involvement, thus making his recovery a long, drawn-out process. In February of 1919 he still had not resumed his normal schedule. The devastating illness had left him in extremely poor physical condition: "What bones are they that rub together so unpleasantly in the middle of you in extreme emaciation?"[3]

Some accounts of the pandemic have suggested that the disease disappeared mysteriously on New Year's Day, 1919.[4] This was hardly true, since from early December until the end of January, epidemic disease raged in Shansi, China, the same province where the so-called pneumonic plague had erupted the year before. The current Shansi epidemic was as infectious and as fatal as that in 1917-18. According to Dr. Percy T. Watson of Fenchow, the mortality rate was a horrific one hundred percent. Moreover, eighty percent of those who came in contact with victims had caught the disease. Although all factors seemed to point to pneumonic plague again, Plague Commission experts called in to investigate found no plague bacilli. A microscopic examination of the pathological specimens taken from one of the fatalities seemed to show a similar picture to that found in the pneumonias and pulmonary edemas accompanying the epidemic of Spanish influenza. What then was the epidemic in Fenchow and Linhsien County? The doctor frankly did not know—influenza was not supposed to be such a fatal disease.[5]

In Paris another wave of influenza took hold as the winter progressed. On February 18 health authorities in the French capital announced that the number of deaths from the disease or its complications for the previous three weeks had been, respectively, 284, 370, and 550.[6] Many Americans in France during the early months of 1919 succumbed to the pandemic disease. Among them: General Pershing's personal aide-de-camp, Representative William P. Borland of Kansas City, Kansas, age fifty-one, a member of Congress for ten years who had been defeated in the 1918 primary

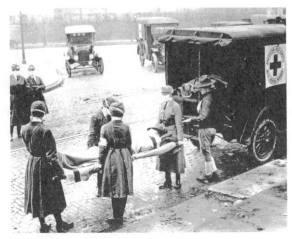

22. Red Cross Motor Corps on duty in Saint Louis

elections; and, Colonel Carl Boyd, age forty, of Adamsville, Georgia. In London, Admiral W. S. Sims, commander of the American fleet in the Atlantic, also lost his aide-de-camp, Commander Edward G. Blakeslee, a thirty-one year-old Annapolis graduate. All three died of pneumonia.[7]

Congressman Borland was the third United States Representative to succumb to the pandemic. Only one, Jacob E. Meeker of St. Louis, Missouri, had died at the height of the autumn wave of the disease. His death had drawn national attention when he had married his private secretary in a death-bed ceremony only hours before his passing.[8] Three months later, on January 25, 1919, Pennsylvania's Representative Edward Robbins became the second congressional fatality in Sommerset, Pennsylvania, where he had gone to make an address and died after only a few days' illness.[9]

The diplomatic corps, American and foreign, also continued to pay their dues to flu as the new year began. By October 20, the *Washington Post* had already reported deaths at the Argentine, Japanese, and British embassies, and among the Chinese, Haitian, and Dominican legations. In November came the announcement of the death in London of the Secretary of the American Embassy at Rome, Thomas Hinckley. And, on January 10, 1919, the Cuban legation in Washington reported it had suffered its second fatality in two weeks. Within another fortnight the American Consul at Guadalajara, Mexico, was dead of a post-influenzal embolism. There was no clear-cut abatement of the pandemic as 1919 came in.[10]

On the contrary, some New England towns near Boston found it necessary to close their schools and recreation centers again as the new year began. Coast Guard stations in Rhode Island were virtually out of commission for some time after Christmas and eighteen thousand pupils were absent in the Washington, D.C., schools on January 3. Towards the end of January, the *Washington Post* reported the increase of influenza in the Army camp zones was a bafflement to the doctors. Some states were reporting fewer cases, and others more. Medical authorities were wondering if the weather might be affecting the erratic spread of the disease.[11]

Yet the overall character of the disease was somewhat different in early 1919 in that it tended to be highly explosive among those who had come through the fall season unscathed. Children's homes, orphan asylums, prisons, and religious communities—particularly those institutions that had put in place strict quarantine measures in the autumn—were now hit heavily by the disease. One such institution was the State Training School for Girls in New York, where influenza affected nearly all of the 450 inmates during the early months of 1919.[12] Also ill practically simultaneously were all but four of the forty-eight theologians at the Saint Bonaventure Franciscan Monastery in Patterson, New Jersey.[13]

Flu also infected two of the aristocratic sheep that were frolicking on the White House lawn late in January. An expert called in from the Department of Agriculture promptly placed the ailing sheep in an animal hospital. Their usual caretaker, the White House gardener, announced that he expected them to recover within a few days. The sheep had come to graze upon the lawn during the war as an economy measure, and at the same time to make money for the Red Cross, their wool being auctioned off at shearing time to the highest bidder.[14]

Theater managers in Savannah, Georgia, also found January of 1919 no kinder to their bankrolls that the previous months had been. On the fifteenth the "flu ban" went into effect again, with restrictions more rigid than before. This was the third such order in the Georgia community. Amusement places in the southern city had not had two full weeks' business at any time since the first of October. As the weeks went by, the managers and owners of Savannah's theaters asked the court for an injunction against the Mayor, City Council, and Sanitary Board to either get the ban removed or to have a similar proscription put on all other businesses in the city. The legal action probably helped convince the local political and health authorities to call off the ban on February 17. However, school children in Savannah were refused permission to enter the movie houses for an additional five weeks, and the new ruling required that all amusement places had to close between the hours of two and three and six and seven for thorough cleanings. Five months of hard times had befallen the city's entertainment centers.[15]

Death from influenza continued to be no stranger in 1919. Broadway's lights dimmed on the evening of January 14 to show respect for the promising young actor, Shelley Hull, who had died at 6:55 p.m., a victim of influenzal pneumonia. His passing left his actress wife, Josephine Hull (one day to have starring roles in *Arsenic and Old Lace* and *Harvey*), in a state of shock. The influenza which had struck them both early in January had spared the life of only one.[16]

As if influenza fatalities were not enough, the American nation lost one of its most beloved citizens through natural causes on January 6. Death claimed suddenly the darling of the Bull Moosers, former President Theodore Roosevelt, at his Oyster Bay, New York, home. One already depressed influenza victim, upon receiving the news of the demise of his old Progressive leader, reacted undoubtedly as countless other of the former President's followers did. As he lay in bed recovering from influenza, the telephone rang: "Did I know that Roosevelt had died in his sleep the night before?... I was weak with fever. I could only press my face into the pillow and cry like a child. There were many others who wept that day." Tears for a fallen hero and tears for oneself. Nineteen eighteen had been a year of death among family and friends, and now 1919 was beginning on a somber note as well.[17]

Another death to sadden the nation was that of the war hero, Captain Emery Rice, age forty, commander of the S.S. *Mongolia*, which on April 19, 1917, had been the first American ship to sink a German submarine. The *Mongolia* had regularly carried munitions to Great Britain from 1916 to the end of the war. Now, after forty-one wartime voyages across the Atlantic, its captain was dead of influenzal pneumonia, following a week's illness.[18]

For some members of the military, the voyage home to America in early 1919 brought more sickness and death. In mid-February the S.S. *Powhatan* sailed from Bordeaux with more than 2,500 troops on board. Shortly after it had started its journey, an epidemic of influenza erupted and spread so quickly that the captain took the advice of the ship's surgeon and returned to port. There the ailing soldiers were transferred to military hospitals. Some of these troops were unable to get other sailing orders for months.[19]

Fate was crueler to Lieutenant Colonel David Hunter Scott, who contracted influenza while sailing homeward on the *Leviathan*. The thirty-eight-year-old assistant chief of staff of the Twenty-Seventh Division, and son of Major General Hugh L. Scott, the commandant at Camp Dix, New Jersey died of pneumonia in New York's Polyclinic Hospital on March 16.[20] A few days later, Major James A. Roosevelt, age thirty-six, a cousin of the recently deceased Theodore Roosevelt, died on board the S. S. *Great Northern* while the steamship was four hundred miles east of Sandy Hook, New Jersey.[21]

The pandemic also seriously disrupted the work schedules and personal activities of many Americans who participated in the closing events of the war and in the postwar negotiations in Europe that followed the Armistice. At least three men involved with the American Peace Commission died in Paris before the Conference ended and many others were critically ill or incapacitated for days or weeks at a time.

Some Americans who arrived in Europe during the fall and winter of 1918-1919 seemed to have one "cold" after another. In fact, it was said that practically everyone who arrived at the French capital caught the "Paris cold"—or worse. One such victim was statistician Dr. Raymond Pearl, on an assignment for Herbert Hoover's Food Administration. Pearl had left Washington in late October to sail on a ship carrying men, women, children, *and* a thousand soldiers. On board the vessel was the President's daughter, Margaret Wilson, on her way to entertain the troops. Pearl was not impressed with her singing or her beauty: "She is not much account as a singer I would say. If she weren't the President's daughter I think her singing would not take her far. And she sure is homely!"[22] Perhaps Pearl's sour reaction was more the result of his own seasick condition and the terribly bad weather on the crossing. "Damn the Kaiser," he wrote.[23]

Within a few days of his arrival in Paris, Pearl recorded in his diary: "There isn't any doubt that I have a beast of a cold. I have been trying for two days to persuade myself to the contrary, but now I must admit it."[24] He also found that his prior impression that he would be away from the flu epidemic raging in the States had been merely wishful thinking. Paris seemed completely closed up: flu-bound. Pearl now convinced himself that his respiratory ailment was surely not influenza, just one of his old "sneezers." About the third day of his cold, he recorded that he had arisen at 7 a.m. after a "fine sleep and a most thorough sweat." He felt pretty good that morning, despite his cold. The next day, however, he was complaining that his lungs were "pretty sore."[25]

One of the remedies Pearl decided to try for his sore lungs was the open-air treatment. On about the fifth day of his cold, he left his hotel room in the morning for a brisk two-hour walk. Not content with a two-hour treatment, the statistician went out walking again in the afternoon. This time he returned to his room with a very sore tendon on his right foot—in fact, the whole back of his leg was swollen. Pearl decided that he'd be wise to postpone any more "treatments" for a while. The next morning, however, he found his leg was so sore that he was unable to walk at all. Of all days to be so afflicted! Here it was, November 11: "It certainly is hell to be tied up in the house with a bum leg at a time like this."[26] Leg, or no leg, he dragged himself down to the street to join the celebrants as the day progressed.

Many others among those who went abroad to organize and participate in the closing events of the war fared no better than Pearl. In mid-October an important contingent of Americans sailed from New York on the *Northern Pacific*. Colonel Edward M. House was enroute to represent the nation in the Supreme War Council. His party included: his wife; two confidential secretaries; his son-in-law and personal secretary, Gordon Auchincloss; Joseph Grew of the State Department; Frank Cobb of the *New York World*; Navy Surgeon Allen D. McLean (commissioned to look after the health of the party); a few high-ranking Navy officers; and five or six clerical personnel.[27]

Probably the first of the party to catch the Paris cold was Gordon Auchincloss. On October 26 he recorded in his diary that he had had a terrible attack of neuralgia all day, and was therefore afraid he was going to be ill. The next day he had a bad cold and a good deal of neuralgia. On that day, the twenty-seventh, Colonel House had expected General Pershing to stop by. The General cancelled his appointment: he was in bed with influenza. House had to settle for a copy of a cable that Pershing had sent to Washington, which listed his ideas of what the Armistice terms ought to be. The following day, Auchincloss awoke feeling better, but with "a bad cold down rather far in my throat."[28] He was not ill enough, in any event, to be forced to stay in bed.

Two weeks later, on Armistice Day, Auchincloss felt very tired again, and again had a bad cold.[29] He went to the conferences on his schedule, nonetheless. One was with Major Willard Straight, whom House had managed to spirit away from the Army for the purpose of helping to organize the upcoming Peace Commission. Straight, who had been assigned to Marshal Foch's Headquarters, had been the one who had called Colonel House within minutes after the Armistice had been signed. Later on that Armistice Day the Major had traveled into Paris to meet with Auchincloss. The thirty-eight year-old Straight, a former diplomat and Wall Street associate in the House of Morgan, had done a superb job of organizing the War Risk Insurance Bureau's efforts on the Continent the previous winter. Auchincloss and Straight decided that afternoon that the Major's new duties were to be connected with securing accommodations, etc., for the United States' representatives to the Peace Conference.[30]

The man ultimately placed in charge of all arrangements for the American Peace delegation was Joseph Grew, Chief of the Western European Section of the State Department. In appointing Grew on November 13 to be the Secretary General of the American Commission to Negotiate Peace, Secretary of State Robert Lansing made that organization a reality.[31] Straight, Colonel House's appointee, thereupon worked with Grew and Walter Lippmann to develop a detailed plan of operation—the physical arrangements, protocol, agenda—for the Peace Conference. Such a plan was on paper shortly, but before it could be executed, the three men—Grew, Straight, and Lippmann—all came down with influenza.[32]

On November 18, Auchincloss recorded in his diary that Joseph Grew had gone to bed the day before with a fever and every indication that he had influenza. That morning, he wrote, Willard Straight had shown up at the office with a fever of one hundred one and a half—he was promptly sent home to bed. Auchincloss wrote:

"I suppose he has influenza too."[33] On the nineteenth Lippmann and "another man named Hazeltine" were the next victims. Auchincloss sent a secret cable to the State Department informing Under Secretary Frank Polk in Washington of the mounting illness in the organization. He wired Polk that they were working under "serious handicaps."[34] The next day, the twentieth, House's personal secretary noted that not only were Grew and Straight still out of circulation, but that several others, including the Colonel, had colds of varying severity. Another victim was the American ambassador to France, William Sharp. Auchincloss commented: "If this disease spreads we won't have anyone left to do the work."[35]

Colonel House's "cold" turned out to be a serious case of influenza. On the twenty-first a number of American physicians, including Alexander Lambert, John Finney, and Fred Murphy, came in to examine the ailing Colonel. The doctors ordered round-the-clock nursing care immediately. On that same day Auchincloss sent Polk the following telegram:

> Colonel House has requested me to send the following message to you. 'Chief Yeoman Gunner Flodin who was assigned to us by the Navy Department from London office on our arrival and who did for us excellent work died this morning as a result of short illness ending in double pneumonia. Request that you have Secretary of State send personal letter to his family commending his service while detailed to this Mission and expressing deep regret of myself and all those associated with him at his sudden death.'[36]

On the same day Auchincloss, feeling as though he were going to be the next flu victim, dosed himself heavily with aspirin "to knock out the symptoms." It evidently worked. Meanwhile, some of the victims began to show up at work again: Lippmann in a few days, and Grew after about a week. But Willard Straight developed pneumonia. Auchincloss recorded on the twenty-third that while Grew, though weak, was getting better, Sir William Wiseman, formerly of the British Embassy in Washington and now British-American liaison officer in Paris, was on the list of the ailing. Auchincloss wrote: "It is the most depressing atmosphere I have ever been in. Everyone around seems to have something the matter with them."[37]

Within the next week, the medical condition of Colonel House showed some improvement, but that of Willard Straight did not. The entourage of physicians caring for the Colonel now began to look after the Major. When Straight's temperature rose to an ominous 103 degrees on the twenty-third, Auchincloss decided to notify the State Department of his condition, but suggested that the Department withhold the news from Mrs. Straight.[38] On the twenty-fifth, Auchincloss went over to the Hotel Crillon and found the Major in grave condition. Nursing the critically ill, semi-conscious man was his long-time family friend, Daisy Harriman. That very day, Mrs. Harriman decided to send off a cable to Herbert Croly in New York City, informing him that Straight had influenzal pneumonia.

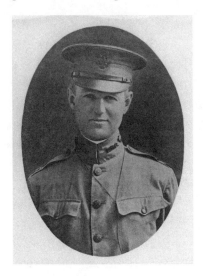

23. Willard Straight, investment banker, diplomat and founder of *New Republic* magazine, in France, 1915.

Would Croly relate this first information of her husband's illness to Dorothy Straight? Mrs. Harriman would keep Croly informed of Straight's condition.[39]

On November 30, Colonel House got out of bed for the first time in ten days and held a fifteen minute conference with French Premier Georges Clemenceau. House wrote the following in his diary for that day:

Today is the first day I have taken up my official work in person for over a week. I have had influenza ten days and have been exceedingly miserable. I never had such care. The Red Cross evidently seized this opportunity to reciprocate for what I have tried to do for that organization. They sent three nurses to take eight hour shifts, and they sent one doctor after another to aid dear Doctor McLean who was with me night and day. So many people have died since this epidemic has scourged the world. Many of my staff have died and poor Willard Straight among them....[40]

Willard Straight died during the early morning hours of December 1. A few hours later, the Colonel sent Mrs. Straight a cable through the State Department, expressing his deepest sympathy on the death of her husband: "His untimely death had deprived his country of one destined to play an important part in moulding her future and I personally feel that I have lost a very dear friend."[41]

Auchincloss thereupon cabled Polk that since Straight's death had occurred after the Armistice, while he was attached to a diplomatic mission, the War Department ought to grant permission for his remains to be shipped back immediately to the United States. Straight's widow decided, however, that her husband should be buried in France with the rest of his fallen comrades. The funeral service was in the American Church in Paris with Bishop Charles H. Brent, Chief of the Chaplain Service, G.H.Q., A.E.F., conducting the rites. According to Daisy Harriman, the men who walked behind

Straight's flag-draped coffin up the Champs Élysées that morning were from all the ranks. Inside the Church the mourners were joined in singing the "Battle Hymn of the Republic" and "Onward Christian Soldiers." From the church the funeral cortege went on to Suresnes, the United States Military Cemetery outside of Paris, for the interment. It was a sorrowful day for the many friends of the winsome young Major.[42]

Meanwhile, the illness of Colonel House was a matter of concern back in Washington. The *New York American* noted on November 23 that his attack of influenza might be more serious than it appeared on the surface. The Colonel was not a robust man, for a sunstroke had previously weakened his heart. The paper recalled that when House had had influenza in March of 1918, he had been confined to his home for two weeks. He then had had a relapse, and spent three additional weeks in bed at the White House. Consequently, the Colonel's current health worried the President. It was particularly unfortunate that Colonel House was sick at this critical juncture in the organization of the Peace Commission.[43]

Some years later, the British newsman, Henry Wickham Steed, reminisced about the failings of Versailles. (Steed was a fan of Colonel House, but not of Woodrow Wilson.) In *Through Thirty Years* he wrote:

> But one serious misfortune—which proved to be a disaster—befell the Conference through the illness of Colonel House. A severe attack of influenza incapacitated him for any work during this critical formative period. Consequently, his guiding influence was absent when it was most sorely needed; and, before he could resume his activities, things had gone too far for him to mend.[44]

House did not regain his health rapidly. Consequently, his physicians refused to let him go to Brest to meet with President Wilson and the other men who, along with himself, would be the official American delegates to the Peace Conference: Secretary of State Robert Lansing; General Tasker H. Bliss; and diplomat Henry White. Also accompanying the President on the *George Washington*, which had left Hoboken, New Jersey on December 4, were more than one hundred men and women who would be serving in various technical, advisory, or organizational capacities at the Conference. Included in this group were twenty-three members of the "Inquiry," an advisory unit made up of historians and other American experts in foreign affairs.[45] Two of the Inquiry staff, Yale historian Charles Seymour and economist Clive Day, had the habit of recording matters of health as well as political events in their journals and letters home. Their writings make clear that sickness, sometimes recurrent, was a common problem among the various delegations at the Conference.

Both Seymour and Day noted that the President had come on board the *George Washington* with a nasty cold. He had consequently remained pretty much out of sight for the first few days of the journey.[46] Accompanying the President, of course, was his personal physician, Rear Admiral Cary T. Grayson. It was while the President was nursing his cold that the movie, "His Second Wife," was featured. Luckily for the recently remarried President, he missed hearing the half-suppressed gasp that rose from the audience when the title flicked across the screen. By the time the vessel landed at the French port on December 14, the President appeared to have recovered completely from his cold.[47]

More than one historian has written that between the arrival of the American group on December 14 and the opening of the Peace Conference on January 18, 1919, the situation was apparently one of utter confusion. Much of the blame was supposedly the President's—his unwillingness to take people, even House, into his confidence. In addition, controversy and petty jealousies arose among the delegates and various groups.[48] Compounding the confusion was the arrival sometime in January of considerably more American personnel—including: the economic experts Herbert Hoover;

Vance McCormick, Chairman of the War Trade Board; Edward N. Hurley, Chairman of the U.S. Shipping Board; and Bernard M. Baruch, War Industries Board Chairman—each bringing with them their own staff assistants. Norman Davis, Samuel Gompers, David Hunter Miller, Thomas W. Lamont—and scores of other technical and financial advisors—arrived as well.[49]

But, amid the chaos, there was for many the arrival of the "Paris cold." In his Christmas letter to his wife, Clive Day wrote that most of the men had caught cold since arriving in France. None seemed badly off, and he himself, he was happy to report, had avoided it. Nevertheless, he assured her that there were capable Army doctors, whose business it was to look after them, at the Hotel Crillon, the headquarters of the American delegation. Since the hotel had steam-heated rooms, if a cold did develop he would be able to nurse it properly. Day reported to his wife that Colonel House was still feeling poorly, but neglected to mention that his own room-mate, Charles Seymour, was not well. Seymour's cold, which had come upon him on the twentieth, was not so serious as to keep him abed. Yet a week later the historian still had the cold in his system, enough so that he had been avoiding as many diplomatic interviews as possible. As the old year ran out, he was still attempting to "kill" his cold.[50]

Rather than killing the cold, Seymour undoubtedly passed it along to Day, who reported on the twenty-ninth: "I seem to be catching the prevalent cold."[51] A week later, January 5, 1919, Day wrote home that his cold seemed to be "passing off quickly without any sequelae, as I believe they are called."[52] But then on January 16 Day wrote that he had been in bed for the last few days. He suspected that his present attack had an influenza element in it, bronchial influenza, perhaps. The Naval surgeon, who had been in to see him in the afternoon, had told him he had a grippy cold, not bronchitis and not influenza, and that he would be fine after a few days in bed. The surgeon had told him that a considerable proportion of Americans arriving in Paris were affected in a similar fashion. Day declared that he liked the Navy doctor better than the healthy, young military surgeon who had been in the day before and who had seemed to lose interest in the case when he found his patient was not spitting blood.[53]

Day probably had influenza, as indicated by his own description of his ailment on January 20:

I was in bed most of the time from Tuesday to Sunday, feeling pretty wretched (with temperature going up to 101 ½) for the first two days. It was unlike any cold I have had, for it did not touch my throat or head, and did not seriously affect my lungs. I coughed one night, but very little since then. Now I feel rather dragged out, and not keen to exert myself, but my head is clear and I have only the trace of a cough or other evidence of inflammation anywhere. I was at work today, moving my desk nearer to the stove....[54]

Day's illness resulted in the cancellation and rescheduling of numerous meetings and interviews. His retreat from everyday activities, however, had much less of an impact upon the Peace Conference than did the second forced retirement of Colonel House in mid-January. Late on the eleventh, House was attacked with pains and chills, resulting in a quick call for medical help. The next morning his temperature climbed to 102 degrees.[55] On January 21 House discussed his own illness in his diary: "Just when the momentum was at its highest and the peace organization was being perfected, I fell ill with a painful attack of kidney trouble."[56] He was able, ten days later, to take up the thread of affairs again, although he still kept to his room. The President had called him almost daily. But he wrote: "It was impossible for me to attend the opening session of the Peace Conference. Everyone regretted this more than I."[57]

For the following week or so, people, including the President, went to visit House. As he attempted to overcome a new siege of the illness, he found himself reading notices of his death coming in from a number of German newspapers. He could not understand how the report of his death had won such wide credence. In any event, he thought the obituary notices were "all too generous." "Bernstorff," he wrote "is particularly complimentary and even so fierce a Prussian as von Reventlow speaks of my demise with deep regret."[58] Back in the United States, the *New York Telegram* also made him front-page news on January 14: "Col House is Reported Dead Abroad… Unconfirmed Rumor …Has Been Ill for Several Weeks in France." A four-by-six inch photograph of the Colonel accompanied the write-up.[59]

The oft-repeated obituary notice prompted the Louisville (Kentucky) *Courier Journal* to make the following comment:

Colonel House: Down on Monday, worse on Tuesday, same on Wednesday, 'tolable' Thursday, up on Friday, dead on Saturday, better on Sunday. The Colonel ain't no Solomon Grundy.[60]

A week later, on January 20, the Washington D.C. *Evening Star* reported that the precarious health of Colonel House was menacing the strength of the American representation at the Peace Conference, and it therefore might be necessary to name a few more official delegates. The talk in Washington was that the new men might be former President William H. Taft and diplomat Elihu Root. With President Wilson due to return to the United States and an ailing Colonel House, a tremendous burden had fallen on the three other representatives, Lansing, White, and Bliss. Additional appointments were not made, however.[61]

While many Americans knew of House's illness, probably few were aware of the number of other Americans at the conference battling illness. The group of economic specialists who had arrived in January had promptly succumbed. On the twenty-second, David Miller felt miserable and was put under a physician's care.[62] Five days later Auchincloss sent a cable to Frank Polk in the State Department informing him that the Treasury Department's Norman H. Davis was ill with influenza, complicated by a touch of pneumonia.[63] Vance McCormick recorded in his diary on January 28 that he had gone to bed early, feeling poorly. Three days later he wrote that he was "still feeling under the weather." Nonetheless he met with Bernard Baruch in Norman H. Davis's room, where Davis was recovering from his pneumonia. On February 2, McCormick noted he had had breakfast with Baruch, but "very late due to oversleeping on account of a bad cold."[64]

The following Sunday, February 9, McCormick and Henry Gross went to see Brigadier General Frank McCoy, who was convalescing from pneumonia in the hospital.[65] A week later, Thomas W. Lamont wired home to his partner Dwight W. Morrow that he was "in the harness after a few days of influenza."[66] Also sick in bed in early February were H. Wickham Steed and Charles Seymour.[67] On February 8, Seymour wrote home to his family in New Haven: "It has been the busiest week of my life. I have had a cold which kept me in bed for a day…"[68] More depressing than the cold, however, was the loss of his aide, Clarence W. Mendell, another Yale man, who had sailed for New York on the eighth, a little over two weeks after being notified that his wife, Katherine, had died of pneumonia on January 21.[69]

Seymour's bout with his cold was not a thing of the past. On February 12 economist Clive Day wrote: "Charlie is in bed today, nursing a cold so as to be ready for the Rumanian affair. He promises to be all right, and I'm lost if he isn't, for I should be quite incompetent to defend his line by myself."[70] Unfortunately for Day, Seymour was no better the next day, and so Day had to represent him at the Rumanian meeting after all. It seems Seymour had tried the open-air treatment on Sunday, February 9. But the walk in the damp cold had evidently not been the right prescription. On Monday, he had a fever yet again. Most of that week he was in bed, attended to, it would appear, by the same military surgeon that Clive Day had had in January, the cheerful soul who "asked if you have been spitting blood." The military doctor suggested that Seymour might smoke a few cigarettes—"says it is good for all kinds of sickness."[71]

Lest one think the American delegation was singled out for illness, representatives of other nations sometimes had to postpone meetings because of illness as well. In February, a would-be assassin's bullet temporarily incapacitated Clemenceau. The attack on Clemenceau shocked the Allies, and it resulted in some delay in the top-level meetings of the conference. Observers noted that both Lloyd George and Wilson agreed that "The Tiger," as Clemenceau was known by the French, was limping badly during March and April, the most crucial months of the conference.[72] For Secretary of State Lansing, the delay was probably a welcome respite, for he, too, was not well.[73] By that time, news of the widespread sickness had filtered back to the United States. Auchincloss received a note late in February from an attorney-friend in the State Department with the following comment: "Shaw tells me you are the only man in Paris who has not been sick. Please keep up the good record."[74] (Sick enough, that is, to be kept in bed.)

Late in February, President Wilson, who had sailed from France on the fourteenth, was back in the United States, ready to do battle with an unfriendly Congress and to muster support for his League of Nations. Throughout the winter his health had remained satisfactory, although some observers had noted a facial twitching from time to time.[75] His few weeks in Washington were evidently enough to bring on another cold when he sailed back to Paris in early March. According to his physician, he was quite sick for two or three days at the beginning of the voyage. He soon recovered, however, and appeared well as the presidential party landed at Brest.[76]

During the next few weeks of intensive diplomatic maneuvering, the negotiations among the "Big Four" would be pivotal. The "Big Four" were the United States, Britain, France and Italy. These nations were represented by: President Wilson; Prime Minister of Great Britain, David Lloyd George; French Premier,

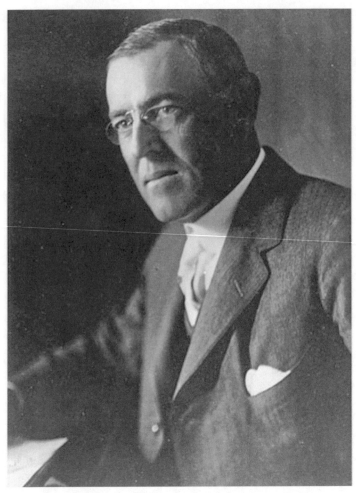

24. President Woodrow Wilson

Georges Clemenceau; and Vittorio Orlando, Prime Minister of Italy. The meetings continued almost daily, and the President appeared very tired at days' end. It was during that time that many of his party fell ill: Mrs. Wilson; her secretary, Edith Benham; Wilson's chief usher, Ike Hoover; and his physician, Cary Grayson.[77] (Daughter Margaret had caught influenza in early February and had been kept in bed at the American Legation in Brussels.)[78] To some observers, the President seemed to grow thin and gray and the twitching became almost continual. He looked tired all the time. Suddenly on April 3 he was ill again, perhaps seriously.[79]

There has always been much controversy about the nature of President Wilson's illness in April of 1919. Both medical and non-medical writers have suggested that the malady was much more serious than influenza. A professor of neurology in New York thought the President probably had a "little stroke," a cerebral vascular occlusion. A less feasible diagnosis, he suggested, was a viral encephalitis or inflammation of the brain, associated with influenza.[80] John Dos Passos wrote some years later that the illness was probably a minor cerebral hemorrhage.[81] According to Gene Smith's *When the Cheering Stopped*, Wilson suffered a thrombosis in his brain, not an attack of influenza.[82] The writers all suggested one thing: the President suffered brain damage in Paris. Consequently, Woodrow Wilson returned from Europe less capable of carrying out the duties of his Presidency.

The President's illness came upon him rather suddenly in the afternoon of April 3, his voice unexpectedly becoming husky during an afternoon meeting. At six o'clock Norman Davis and Vance McCormick found him in bed with a bad cold.[83] The following day Dr. Grayson wired Joseph Tumulty that the "President took severe cold last night." On April 8 Grayson wired that the President was sitting up.[84] Two days later, Dr. Grayson took the time to write a letter to Tumulty describing in greater detail his patient's illness:

> This has been one of the most complexing and trying weeks of my existence here. The President was taken violently sick last Thursday. The attack was very sudden. At three o'clock he was apparently all right; at six he was seized with violent paroxysms of coughing, which were so severe and frequent that it interfered with his breathing. He had a fever of over 103 and a profuse diarrhea. I was at first suspicious that his food had been tampered with, but it turned out to be the beginning of an attack of influenza. That

night was one of the worst through which I have ever passed. I was able to control the spasms of coughing but his condition looked very serious. Since that time he has been gradually improving every day so that he is now back at work—he went out for the first time yesterday. This disease is so treacherous, especially in this climate, and I am perhaps over-anxious for fear of a flare-back—and a flare-back in a case of this kind often results in pneumonia.[85]

There was little doubt in Grayson's mind that President Wilson had had influenza, and certainly the weight of evidence suggests that that was the case. During the President's absence from April 4 until the afternoon of April 8, House found himself at the negotiating table along with Clemenceau and Lloyd George.

Many, including Lloyd George himself, commented on the changes in Wilson's behavior after his illness, some referring to him as having become inattentive, indecisive and forgetful.[86] The President was also to suffer a severe stroke the next September during his fight for American acceptance of the Versailles Treaty.

During the first week in April, influenza and Paris colds were still widespread, especially among the official delegations. While Wilson was in bed, Lloyd George and Colonel House had respiratory ailments. The writer, Lincoln Steffens, himself sick abed on April 8, wrote to a friend that day that he had been down at the Hotel Crillon the day before and "couldn't do much because all the Big Four and some of the little ten were sick."[87] John Dos Passos apparently later forgot that he, too, had been unwell in early April. On April 6, 1919, he wrote to a friend: "I write abed in the last stage of recovery from a remarkable disease, during which a gong rang continually and I coughed in a manner to turn my throat inside out and then outside in again."[88]

At the same time, the American Mission suffered the loss of another of its members to the pandemic disease. According to the New York *Evening Post* for April 8, 1919, Donald Frary of the American Peace Delegation in Paris, was dead at twenty-five.

Frary, who had been a promising young historian at Yale, had been appointed to the Commission at the suggestion of Charles Seymour. He had collaborated with Seymour in the writing of the elder historian's latest book. The younger man, who had had a cold, had visited the French battlegrounds the weekend before his death. On Wednesday he went to bed, the next day to the hospital, even before his friends were aware of his illness. Pneumonia set in on Saturday and he died at noon on Sunday. Seymour wrote: "Pneumonia comes like an accident: two weeks ago he was in perfect health, but he took a chance with his cold."[89]

Because influenza was still taking its toll, April in Paris was a sickly and somber time for the American Peace Commission. Everyone seemed to be tired and irritable—they were living through "strange days."[90] For many of the advisors to the Commission, however, their work was nearing an end. On April 13, Seymour wrote to his New Haven family and friends: "Really this last week has had almost the air of a fin de la saison. No more commission meetings, very few conferences, a great deal of dope as to what was being decided by the Big Four, and a general clearing up of offices."[91] But people were tired rather than elated. It would be a relief to be home again, away from the miserable weather and the "Paris cold."

By the time Seymour and his wife, who had joined him in February, returned to the United States in late spring, the major wave of the pandemic was over. U.S. Public Health authorities later concluded that the pandemic wave that had begun in the fall of 1918, had persisted for thirty-one weeks instead of the expected six to fourteen.[92] The mortality rate for influenza and pneumonia remained above the norm from September 15, 1918, until April 19, 1919. Generally, rates along the east coast fell to within the normal range faster than they did in the midwest. Ohio cities, for instance, had new peaks of high mortality in March of 1919. While Boston's excess monthly death rates per 100,000 for the first four months of 1919 were, respectively, +827, +224, +23, and -42, those in some of the Ohio cities were:[93]

	Cincinnati	Cleveland	Columbus	Dayton
January	+52	+464	+117	+97
February	+523	+413	+215	+96
March	+793	+543	+585	+256
April	+60	+228	+103	+59

As the number of new cases of influenza and pneumonia continued to fall, concern about another disease rose. Early in January 1919, American readers learned that another new mysterious disease, similar to infantile paralysis, was now affecting Europeans. Doctors were calling the disease "lethargic encephalitis," and by March, the disease was on the American side of the Atlantic. The *New York Times* revealed on March 16 that forty "coma" cases, with two deaths, had already occurred in the city. Then, two days later came the report of two deaths in New England and another in Richmond, Virginia. According to physicians at the Beth Israel Hospital in New York, the disease had a tendency to follow influenza. About half of the cases treated at the New York hospital were apparently post-influenzal complications; the other cases were probably "true epidemic coma." Lethargic encephalitis was a grave disease, for many of the victims were dying.[94]

Perhaps the spring of 1919 might have been a more cheerful time had the newspapers been less assiduous about reminding people that disease was still taking its toll. The casualty lists from Europe, even in May, were a daily reminder that November 11 brought no end to sorrow. The figures released by the War Department at the end of April showed a total of 111,179 military deaths had occurred since the beginning of the war. More than half of the deaths, 56,532, or fifty-one percent, had been the result of disease. Significantly, 12,000 of the disease-related deaths had occurred after the cessation of hostilities in November.[95]

In August of 1918, author John Jay Chapman, whose sister Eleanor had recently lost her son in the war, wrote the following observations to his father:

> *When you lose a boy in the war and at a time everyone else is losing them and it's part of the age and of value to the country—this is very different from having one die of disease in ordinary times—and there's a natural law which alleviates the grief. Otherwise it would be intolerable. Everyone would be in despair.*[96]

The pandemic-related deaths may have been of no value to the country, but they certainly were "part of the age." Perhaps Thomas Wolfe summed up the grief, and sometimes bitterness, so many people felt as the pandemic took away their loved ones. In *Look Homeward, Angel*, pandemic influenza passed by the cancer-ridden Gant only to claim the youthful Ben. The Gants, Wolfe wrote, "all felt the grim trickery of Death, which has come in by the cellar as they waited at the window."[97] Wolfe's family had expected death to claim the long-ill head of the household, not a son in his twenties.

Fate, in the form of the flu, had played a cruel trick on too many American families. For widows like Josephine Hull, there was no natural law to alleviate their grief, and in their desperation many turned to charlatans who promised communication with their departed ones. America became a nation in mourning, a nation with a new consciousness of the impact of disease.

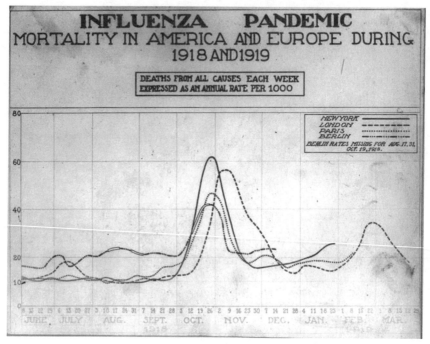

Figure 5.1 Influenza pandemic mortality in America and Europe during 1918 and 1919.

6

The Aftermath (1919)

But poverty is not merely a cause of sickness; it is also a result of sickness. Sickness is so intimately related to destitution that it is often impossible to determine whether it is a cause or an effect.[1]

If these words reflected the distressful situation of those at the bottom of the economic ladder in the United States at the beginning of 1918, how much more meaningful the words were in 1919, following the influenza pandemic. The pandemic had a noticeable impact on both individual lives and on human institutions. It forced the government to take up the questions of support for medical research and of the relationship between public health and private medicine. There was a remarkable institutional response to the pandemic, which will be examined in this chapter. But the institutional response grew out of the desperate needs of individual victims of the pandemic. Social workers and others began to see how essential it was that communities provide certain minimum services necessary to safeguard the health of their citizens. Health matters would have to become a public rather than a private concern.

Prior to the fall of 1918, destitution had all too often been equated with ignorance and lack of industry. But the pandemic provided ammunition to those, who like Lillian Wald, had been pleading for years that poverty was a more complicated phenomenon. Charity was often not the answer for the destitute. Yet in the wake of the pandemic, charity was usually the only avenue open to help the hundreds of thousands of flu victims. In fact, the families selected for the "Hundred Neediest Cases" in New York City were probably the fortunate poor. Charitable organizations saw that the destitute families so chosen returned to normal life, if possible. In the case of John M. referred to in Chapter 4, the *New York Times* reported on May 18, 1919, that his family was once again self-supporting. Although John had recovered from his influenza in due course, the doctors, fearing that he might develop tuberculosis, had refused to let him return to work until mid-April. During the many months of convalescence at home, John and his family had received an adequate diet from the Brooklyn Bureau of Charities. By mid-May, the family was happy and healthy once again.[2]

Case #36, also referred to earlier, describing a family situation where the father had died having an appendectomy following influenza, was still being overseen by the same charitable organization in May. Every member of the family had had influenza following the father's death and each had received emergency medical treatment and a referral to the local health center for follow-up care. When doctors at the center had recommended milk and eggs for three of the children, they were provided. As of May, the Bureau was considering sending the widow and her children back to her relatives in Italy, provided conditions on the other side were favorable for a decent existence.[3]

In another case previously unmentioned, three members of a poverty-stricken family had had influenza after the Christmas season. The same Brooklyn agency had placed the ailing children in a convalescent home. After two weeks the youngsters returned to their homes, and were later reported to be "doing good work at

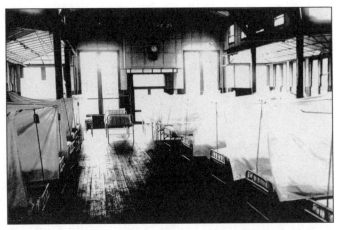

25. Interior of house used for influenza victims by the Red Cross in New Haven, Connecticut, 1919

school." Care such as these three families had received was sorely needed throughout the New York City area.[4]

More fortunate were the needy in Cincinnati, where the social agencies joined together in the aftermath of the pandemic to care for any and all of the community's victims desiring assistance. According to the President of the American Public Health Association (APHA), Dr. Lee K. Frankel of Metropolitan Life, Cincinnati was "doing the first piece of real [restorative] work of any city in the country."[5]

In an address read before the general sessions of the APHA in New Orleans on October 28, 1919, Cincinnati's Health Commissioner, Dr. William H. Peters, told the audience of his city's crusade to fight disease. The Cincinnati Health Officer began his report by remarking on the considerable scientific research inspired by the pandemic. Nationwide a "small army of scientific investigators" had joined in an all-out effort to find the "cause and mode of transmission" of influenza. Yet little had been done for the victims of the disease. As Dr. Peters noted, certain phrases: "I'm not feeling right," "I haven't my usual pep," and "I'm all in since I had the flu," had become commonplace expressions. It was the doctor's opinion that few influenza victims had escaped without pathologic changes. Besides the physical complications and sequelae, however, were others much less apparent:

> Shattered homes, health and income, inability to work, impaired efficiency, loss of earning power, and mental anxiety and distress, coupled with the high cost of living, completed the chain of horrors following the ravages of the epidemic.[6]

Cincinnati, as mentioned earlier, had had a new breakout of influenza in the early months of 1919. Beginning with September 1918, and ending with May 1919, the excess monthly death rates (annual basis) per 100,000 from influenza and pneumonia in the Ohio city were, respectively, +18, +2,140, +1,285, +1,520, +52, +523, +793, +60, and -28. Obviously, February and March of 1919 continued to bring many deaths to the Ohio community.[7]

According to Dr. Peters, it was not until February 1919 that the city's social agencies became aware of the serious economic effects of the pandemic. Institutions caring for dependent children were by then hard-pressed to find places for those needing care, and the Mothers' Pension Department required additional funding to help the scores of women who had lost husbands as the winter progressed. In addition, the Cincinnati Associated Charities learned that more than fifty percent of the wage earners in four hundred dependent families "had been unable to return to work, either because of their physical condition or because their positions had been filled by others during their absence on account of illness."[8]

The increase in the number of applications for assistance resulted in a rapid depletion of budgeted funds in the various social agencies. In consequence, a group of local citizens reported the drain of local funds to the Cincinnati War Chest, with the recommendation that a special fund be set up to aid influenza victims. In the end, the Board of Directors of the Cincinnati Red Cross decided to finance the effort to provide "medical care, nursing service, and material relief" to the city's sick. To the so-called "American Red Cross Health Crusade," the local Red Cross War Chest appropriated fifty thousand dollars, half for the medical division, and half for relief.[9]

The medical plan put into operation divided the city into thirteen districts, each containing a central health station. At each school-based health station was a team of three: physician, nurse, and clerical assistant. The primary aim of the team was to diagnose disease with patients then being sent to their family physicians, to district doctors, or to hospitals or clinics, depending on the nature of their medical problems and ability to pay. The stations were theoretically not designed to treat flu victims. Yet in cases where instruction, supervision, and perhaps a tonic were needed, such patients were often carried along for a month or two. On hand at the health stations were considerable supplies of medicinal remedies: malt and cod liver oil; syrup hydriotic acid; syrup iron iodide; saccharated carbonate of iron; and other simple remedies for the children and asthenic adults.[10] "Asthenics" were run-down and under-nourished persons needing tonics, proper diets, and rest.

When the schools opened in September, four months after the stations had begun to function, the health centers became night clinics. Within that time, the health crusaders had listed 13,772 influenza victims, examined 7,058, and found 5,624 (nearly eighty percent) in need of some sort of medical assistance. Statistics revealed a surprisingly high number of cardiac cases (643) among the category "Defects and Diseases." Most of the patients showing cardiac irregularities had fallen ill during the October wave of the pandemic. Fortunately, however, few showed organic heart disease. On the other hand, Cincinnati medical authorities had been struck by the extraordinary number of prominent citizens who had died suddenly, apparently of heart attacks, during the early months of 1919. Inquiries showed that many had had influenza during the pandemic. Could there be a connection, physicians wondered?[11]

Also on the increase in the months following the protracted epidemic was the number of new victims of tuberculosis. Those seen in the four-month period in the Cincinnati health stations amounted to 183.[12] Many pale, sickly-looking individuals who proved not to be tubercular were diagnosed as "asthenics." One group of Cincinnati doctors who were considerably busier in this period were the "nose and throat" specialists. Health station physicians sent them 190 patients for tonsillectomies and adenoidectomies. (At the time, the tonsils were suspected to be a probable source of infection.) Of course, another group kept busy during the summer months were the radiologists, who made 449 plates from 174 patients.[13] At the end of the four months, the Health Crusade's medical division had used almost eighteen thousand dollars of its twenty-five thousand dollar appropriation. The residual seven thousand dollars would pay for the night clinics, educational publicity, and, if necessary, help those needing material assistance.[14]

The relief section of the Cincinnati Red Cross Health Crusade did not hold its first organizational meeting until May 26, 1919. At the onset the Relief Committee planned to hire its own case investigators, but soon found that was going to be a prohibitively costly operation. Instead, the Committee decided to work through the existing charitable organizations in the city: the Associated Charities, the Bureau of Catholic Charities, and the United Jewish Charities. Requests for material assistance henceforth came from the investigators of those agencies, and were then acted upon by the Relief Committee. However, the Committee ordinarily withheld its funds, except in emergency situations, until the patient or applicant had seen a physician at one of the health stations or a private practitioner. Generally the Relief Committee required a written diagnosis from the attending physician before acting on the case. Then the Committee, in consultation with the doctor, made out an individual budget for each person or family to be assisted.[15]

Relief was primarily given to influenza victims. Those widowed during the pandemic and who had no means of support received a "full budget." In cases where the Relief Committee funds were insufficient to pull the family through the crisis, the applicants were referred to the city's usual relief-giving agencies. When the Health Crusade took an influenza victim under its wing, the whole family received attention. Malnourished and sickly individuals were examined, and a "plan worked out for health betterment," even though such family members may not have had influenza.[16]

The Relief Committee also attempted to help those who were still unable to return to a normal work schedule. Light duties were found for numerous flu victims, at a lower rate of pay, of course, but with a sufficient amount of relief provided so that the families were able to manage. In other cases where rest at home was indicated, the victims received a greater budgetary allocation. The Committee sent still other individuals to convalescent homes, or boarded them in the country if the doctor thought fresh air might be conducive to a speedy recovery.[17]

For healthy widows with three children or fewer, the Committee found part-time employment, perhaps two or three days a week. In such cases, the Relief group also made arrangements for the care of the dependent children. In some situations, families received money to travel to the homes of relatives living in other parts of the nation, if they would assume financial responsibility for the victimized families. Still other families received food instead of money. When doctors prescribed special or supplemental diets, items such as milk and eggs, the Committee purchased and distributed them.[18]

By the fall of 1919, the Cincinnati American Red Cross Health Crusade's Relief Committee was expending approximately one thousand dollars a week to one hundred and fifty families. But the allocation of funds was only half of the plan to help the poor: "It is our aim to reconstruct socially each family, as far as that is possible, by the time the patient is well physically, so that the case when dismissed is cured in the highest sense of the term."[19] The Health Crusaders wanted both better public health and good citizens. The

Relief Committee and the Medical Section were confident that influenza survivors in the city who had needed help had received it. Committee members also believed that the Crusade had prepared the people for the expected fall drive of influenza, which would be turned into a "brilliant counter-offensive."[20]

The Cincinnati American Red Cross Health Crusade represented a distinct change in what was considered to be the proper realm for Red Cross activities. Prior to and during the influenza pandemic, the American National Red Cross had functioned as an agency providing emergency medical assistance, rarely involving itself in social welfare-related work. Red Cross monies had been used to pay for salaries of nursing personnel and for medical supplies required during emergency situations. During the autumn wave of the pandemic the Red Cross had assigned and remunerated, in less than two months, fifteen thousand nursing personnel: enrolled nurses, Home Defense nurses, student nurses, practical nurses, and lay women.[21]

Enrolling women into the ranks of the Red Cross during the pandemic had proved to be a more difficult task than its officers had perhaps anticipated. Because trained personnel were in such short supply, there was often keen competition for their services. Private citizens, in some instances, had offered nurses twenty-five to fifty dollars per month more than the Red Cross was authorized to pay.[22] Such wages were quite an enticement at a time when nurses usually earned about seventy dollars per month. But if there were nurses who had considered their pocketbooks first, there were other dedicated women who had worked around the clock for an average day's pay. And, in many communities, women had simply volunteered their services for free during the height of the autumn wave of the disease.

Because the Red Cross had rapidly depleted its funds in the fall of 1918, division directors of Civilian Relief had received reminders that the Home Service sections must confine themselves exclusively to soldiers' and sailors' families, their proper province.

The Red Cross was not to "assume administrative responsibilities or commit [the] Red Cross to any relief expenditures whatever." Only where existing social agencies were unable to handle the situation would they assign temporary personnel to do relief work.[23] Many local chapters, however, did set up Emergency Influenza Committees during the height of the pandemic and often used whatever funding they had available for both medical and social relief.

The Red Cross's wish to stay out of the civilian relief problem vanished, as early 1919 brought no end to the pandemic. On March 1, 1919, the General Manager of the Red Cross in Washington, D.C., sent a memo to the division managers on the subject of "Home Service for Victims of Influenza." The Red Cross had decided to authorize the Home Service sections to extend assistance "to families whose distress is manifestly due to the epidemic," in communities lacking suitable agencies to undertake the services needed.[24] Local divisions would be allowed to use funds set aside for the Home Service and "any other unappropriated funds now in the

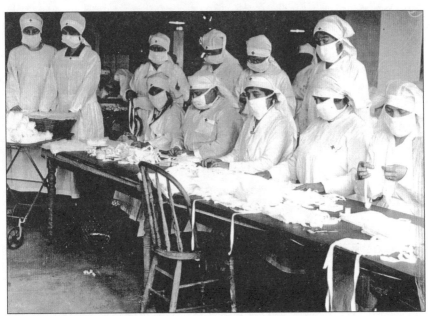

26. Red Cross workers in Boston making masks for protection against influenza, 1919.

chapter treasury."[25] In this way, cities such as Cincinnati were able to provide more help to the victims of the pandemic.

As a result of the influenza pandemic, the public became aware of two vital health-related needs. One was the necessity for organized public health nursing in every community, and the other concerned health education. In December 1918, Louis J. Frank, the Superintendent of New York's Beth Israel Hospital, wrote letters to former Presidents Roosevelt and Taft, to the Surgeons General of the Army, Navy, and Public Health Service, and to other prominent Americans urging that in the post-war period Congress ought to enact a law for the "universal training of females in nursing." He suggested that since women had gained equal rights, they had acquired some "equal duties of service." Unfortunately, the public school system neglected to teach young women matters of health—knowledge of paramount importance for the future mothers of America. The Beth Israel Superintendent noted that because the nation's hospitals could accommodate two million student nurses, why not require all girls at the age of sixteen to spend two years in theoretical and practical nurse training? The problem, he thought, was particularly critical, given the shortage of trained nurses to care for the illnesses related to demobilization.[26]

Although Superintendent Frank's appeal went unanswered, public health nursing grew remarkably in the post-war era. One of the first important steps was to create, in addition to the Army and Navy Nurse Corps, a third government nurse corps, that of the United States Public Health Service. That move began in December of 1918, when Surgeon General Rupert Blue appealed to the Red Cross Nursing Service for additional nurses. At the same time, Blue appointed on a temporary basis Lucy Minnigerode, an executive nurse, to tour the Public Health Service's Marine Hospitals. Following the inspection tour, Blue gave her a desk in his office. Then, when Congress passed Public Act 326 on March 3, 1919, making the Public Health Service the medical agency responsible for the care of the military's sick and disabled, Miss

Minnigerode was appointed superintendent of the U.S. Public Health Service's Nursing Service. By the end of the fiscal year 1920, the Nurse Corps of the Public Health Service numbered 1,100 nurses.[27]

Public Health Nursing in the United States began a new phase in 1918 when the Rockefeller Foundation called together a group of fifty people to discuss the problem of educational requirements for the profession. Chairman of the conference was Yale Professor of Public Health Charles-Edward A. Winslow. In March 1919, the President of the Foundation appointed a Committee for the study of Public Health Nursing Education, and in 1920 the scope of its study widened to include nursing education as a whole. From this committee came Josephine Goldmark's classic report, "Nursing and Nursing Education in the United States." Published in 1923—some fifty years after the founding of the first new Nightingale schools of nursing—the Goldmark report gave birth to endowments for university schools of nursing that provided the foundation for the beginning of truly professional nursing education in this country.[28]

In addition to the efforts carried out at the national level, some American communities began to organize their own public health nursing agencies as well. Rochester, New York, provides an example. In that city, the influenza pandemic brought to the attention of its citizens the "inadequate outdoor nursing service" (sometimes called a "Visiting Nurse Service"). As a result of the joint efforts of the Social Workers' Club and other Rochester agencies employing nurses, a well-known public health nurse went to the city with the idea of coordinating the various nursing services into one central agency. The result was the organization of the Public Health Nursing Association, and a four-month course of study prescribed for those who wished to work as public health nurses in that city.[29]

Rochester's new public health curriculum, called the "Family and Community Standards for Public Health Workers," included formal lectures, study of case records, and field work. As of the fall of 1919, the Rochester work was being financed by the

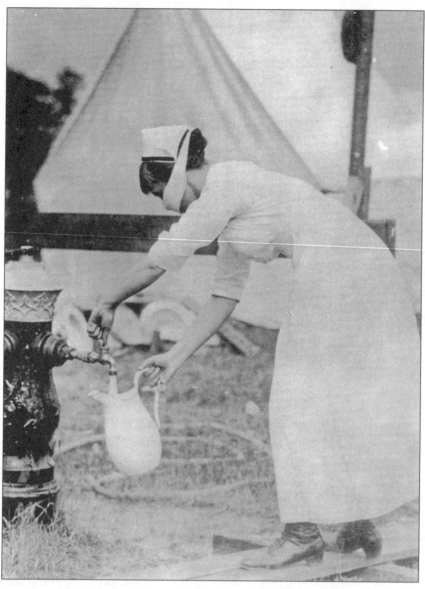

27. Nurse wearing a mask for protection against influenza, 1918

Third Presbyterian Church, which offered, in addition to the public health studies, an intensive course in social work for its volunteer staff personnel. The Director of Rochester's Public Health Nursing Association soon ran into problems, however, with the proposed training program. Too many Rochester citizens thought that "we are asking too much in demanding our staff nurses to take this four months' training in the District."[30] Public Health Nursing still lacked solid support as a separate course of study.

The second vital need brought to light by the pandemic was for "health education." In many communities the fear of influenza had been so marked that it had resembled the terror accompanying the Black Plague in the Middle Ages. For example, during the major autumn wave of the pandemic, rumors had spread rapidly across the nation that the U.S. Army was executing nurses and medical officers at the camps who were acting as spies and spreading Spanish influenza among the men. The Acting Surgeon General of the Army, Brigadier General Charles Richard (Surgeon General Gorgas was in Europe), had to issue a statement to the press that the rumors were "insidiously false reports." He had surmised it was a piece of German propaganda.[31] Nevertheless, people had attributed influenza to many causes: the weather; German agents; and poor diets. The pandemic had revealed how little the public knew about communicable diseases and good health. On the other hand, some physicians had not been much better informed. The Dean of Fordham University's Medical School had prescribed the following regimen for influenza: "rest, alcohol, simple diet, and the free use of mustard plasters and hot mustard footbaths."[32]

In early March 1919 the American Red Cross announced that it planned to send thirty to fifty nurses who had recently returned from France to "teach prevention and control of disease" from Chautauqua platforms. In fact, some of the nurses were already speaking on the special Winter Chautauqua Circuit in Florida, trying out the plan. These lecture tours would be an integral part of the Red Cross peace-time operation, and would include subjects such as the "Home fight against infection," and "Can you cook?" Lecturing nurses would proclaim a "gospel of public health, of sanitation, cleanliness, wholesomeness, and happiness."[33]

The Chautauqua circuit catered primarily to an adult audience. To reach children, other strategies were developed and used. New York's Westchester County hired "Cho-Cho, the Health Goblin," whose mission on earth was to "teach children to be happy and healthy."[34] The New York Times for June 8, 1919, featured a picture in its rotogravure section showing Cho-Cho telling nearly a thousand kiddies, who were recent guests of Mr. and Mrs. Frank A. Vanderlip at their home, Beechwood, on the Hudson, "the story of the Lowly Potato, and of its Value as Food." Also in the picture were: the State Commissioner of Education, Dr. John H. Finley; Dr. Emmet Holt from the College of Physicians and Surgeons; and several other adults involved in health education.

Schools and colleges became more health-education and health-maintenance-oriented after the pandemic as well. Some institutions had suspended their health departments during the war years, since so many members of the staff were in military service. On many campuses physical examinations and medical treatment had been the responsibility of the medical divisions of the Army and Navy Student Training Corps. After the war, however, university health departments quickly reorganized as they had been in 1916-17. A comparison of statistics gathered at Yale for the years 1916-17 and 1919-20 showed fewer defective teeth and hypertrophied tonsils in 1919-20, but the greatest change occurred in the category "Heart and Circulation":

Total Examinations	1916-17	1919-20
	1,508	1,359

Functional Murmurs	1916-17 Number	1916-17 Percent	1919-20 Number	1919-20 Percent
	176	11.7	336	24.7

Almost twenty-five percent of the students examined had functional murmurs. Many physicians wondered if the pandemic had caused the increase and realized that these and other students would need to receive more careful health maintenance in the post-war years.[35]

Columbia University responded to the challenge with a new system of physical education. Medical surveillance would be extended to the freshman from the first day on campus until the graduate received his diploma. "The idea," said Health Service chief, Dr. W. H. McCastline, "is not to bring everyman up to the Rooseveltian standard of strenuous life, but to perfect him in his own standard."[36] Army-type records of defects would be kept, with the expectation that problems would be corrected. Columbia hoped to turn out graduates who were one hundred percent physically and mentally sound.

To accomplish this purpose, the university health service set out to devise and implement an effective system of medicine and hygiene that emphasized prevention rather than treatment. Columbia's Dean Hawkes and Dr. McCastline were each of the opinion that physical ailments were often contributing factors for poor work in the classroom. To show this was true, in June 1919, the University planned to apply psychological entrance examinations. It was hoped that information from the examinations would permit university authorities to "have a clear answer to the question why if he [the student] should fall behind in his studies."[37]

Although the U.S. Army had popularized such psychological tests, it may be that the unsettled atmosphere on many campuses in the immediate post-war period influenced the administration to adopt such measures. In New Haven, for instance, Yale President Arthur T. Hadley wrote in his Annual Report for 1918-19 of the conditions during the spring of 1919:

> *In no year has the college spirit been more active, and on the whole more wholesome, than in the spring of 1919. This was manifested under particularly trying circumstances during the last week in May, when crowds of idle men and boys, partly misled by false reports of agitators—the trouble came just at the time when bomb-throwing outrages were most in evidence in other parts of the country—but chiefly actuated by an irresponsible desire for a row, attacked college buildings and society halls and individual students who happened to be separated from their fellows. The self-restraint of the student body, and the wise leadership of Colonel Beard and Dean Jones, turned what might otherwise have proved a public disaster into a victory for law and order.*[38]

On June 3, 1919, the nation's newspapers printed headlines across the top of page one similar to those run in the *New York Times*: "Midnight bombs for Officials in 8 Cities; Bombers Die at Attorney General's House; Two Victims at Judge Nott's House Here; Bombs in Boston, Cleveland, [and] Pittsburgh."[39] It was the beginning of a long, hot summer. It was in this context then, that many collegiate authorities probably thought that psychological testing was a wise precautionary measure—a good "preventive medicine" for identifying problems in the college environment.

Also concerned with preventive measures in the wake of the pandemic were the Community Councils for National Defense. After the war ended there seemed little need for such organizations to continue to function. However, the pandemic provided a reason to keep some of them viable. In early April of 1919, New York City's Community Council discussed the after-effects of influenza and ways to minimize the death rate. Before the meeting adjourned, a Health Committee chaired by Dr. Lee K. Frankel, president of the APHA, came into existence. Its purpose: to establish and implement preventive influenza measures. Dr. Frankel pointed out that following the pandemic of 1891, the death rate had remained abnormally high for about four or five years. Unless rigorous measures were now taken, there would probably be a repetition in the death pattern. The rigorous measures included getting health questions before the people. Dr. Frankel thought the councils could get the message to every resident of every community. He added: "I am now working on a simplified sanitary code that will be easy for everybody to understand, and the organization of Community Councils can bring it to the attention of every individual."[40]

All of the previously-mentioned efforts to prevent a recurrence of the horrors of 1918 supplemented the work of the United States Public Health Service, where officials were attempting to obtain federal funding to permit additional research on influenza. At least four resolutions were introduced into Congress as 1919 progressed.[41] One forwarded to Congress by several section meetings of the American Medical Association during its annual meeting at Atlantic City in June was for an appropriation of $1,500,000 for the Public Health Service to continue its research activities.[42] Along with the resolution, members of the AMA sent a series of questions and answers pertaining to influenza to Congressional members, the last series being:

Q. *The economic loss to the country of the epidemic?*

A. *The economic loss can hardly be estimated. The 500,000 deaths alone represent $2,500,000,000 economic loss. Economists all agree to the fact that $5,000 is the minimum social and economic value of a human life. It is safe to say that 10,000,000 had the disease and that they lost 150,000,000 working days. At a minimum combined loss of wage and production of $7.00 per day, there has been* *another $1,000,000,000 of economic loss to the country. In other words, conservatively speaking, we had between $3,000,000,000 and $4,000,000,000 loss in this last epidemic.*[43]

As Dr. Cushing had noted in the fall of 1918, Congressmen had hearts and pants' pockets. The problem was, however, now that the medical emergency had passed, would they still have "hearts"?

One speaker at the Atlantic City medical sessions suggested another way the nation might profitably spend its money. Dr. W.S. Thayer of the Johns Hopkins Medical School, who had recently returned from war-time service in Europe, told the Congress of American Physicians and Surgeons that the war had shown the value of rehabilitation hospitals. Physicians at the rest camps had become more familiar with the common diseases as well as the more obscure maladies. Experience had shown that in 628 cases of influenza treated at the Army's hospital camps, the average stay was thirty-one days; in 170 pneumonia cases, fifty-eight days; in 233 cases of acute bronchitis, thirty-six days; in 1,195 cases of gas poisoning, thirty-seven days; in 192 cases of concussion, thirty-five days, and in 80 cases of exhaustion, forty days for recovery. Dr. Thayer suggested that the time had come to establish similar "Peace Disease Camps" to treat ailing civilians. He argued that, now that the war in Europe was over, the war against disease had to be won.[44]

But the Battle of the Flu, which had begun in September of 1918, continued to baffle the medical community as 1919 progressed. During the fall of 1918 many physicians had not seemed familiar with either the symptoms or the course of pandemic influenza. Most of the medical profession then believed that the last pandemic had occurred about 1891, more than twenty-five years earlier. Consequently, for doctors less than fifty years of age, diagnosing and treating pandemic influenza was a somewhat new experience.[45]

During the fall of 1918, New York City's Health Commissioner Royal S. Copeland had said that the dangerous character of influenza was its tendency to change into pneumonia. Fortunately, he added, only a small percentage of affected persons developed the second-day pneumonia, which was generally fatal in its results.[46] The course of the disease, if fatal, he said, usually covered seven days: "three days of influenza, two days of normal temperature, two of pneumonia, and the end on the seventh day."[47] But the influenza fatalities actually showed no consistency in the length of time from onset to termination. The prominent epidemiologist, Yale's Dr. Charles-Edward A. Winslow, noted that in a number of cases he had seen people who were perfectly well die within twelve hours of getting sick.[48] Still other influenza victims lived for two weeks or longer after the onset of influenza until dying. Physicians could not agree on just what kind of disease influenza was.

In an effort to solve the influenza mystery, New York's Governor Charles S. Whitman appointed, in mid-October 1918, eighteen nationally prominent physicians and scientists, including Dr. Winslow, to serve on an Influenza Commission. Selected as its chairman was New York State Commissioner of Health, Hermann M. Biggs. The Commission (see Appendix B for the list of members) met in New York City at the Academy of Medicine on October 30, 1918, November 22, 1918, December 20, 1918, and February 14, 1919.[49]

At the first meeting of the Commission, Dr. Biggs noted that in his thirty years of medical experience, there had never been any crisis in which physicians had felt so helpless. Although, he said, "we have all known that influenza was prevailing in Europe for a year," the American medical profession had been completely unprepared to deal with the problem.[50]

One of the first Commission members called upon to relate his experiences during the pandemic was Dr. Henry A. Christian, Professor of Medicine at Harvard University. The Boston physician's remarks pertained to the uncertain relationship between influenza and pneumonia:

> *The most striking thing in Boston that bears on these statistics is all the cases of the seriously sick are cases of pneumonia. I don't believe there is any sense in trying to distinguish the cases who die from influenza without pneumonia from those who die from influenza with some form of pneumonia. In none of the fatal cases have we failed to find definite signs of pneumonia before they died....The experience so far as the autopsy material is concerned is fully borne out with the autopsies they had in the Navy and the Army. I myself doubt whether any appreciable number of individuals have died during this epidemic without pneumonia. Some die in a short time from overwhelming toxemia; even then they have bronchitis or pulmonary pneumonia. Some have cases of meningitis. All the cases of meningitis we have seen have been of epidemic cerebrospinal, or tubercular, or pneumococcus meningitis—no cases apparently of influenza meningitis [the meaning here is a meningitis caused by the influenza bacillus]. It seems to me we may just as well consider this disease a pulmonary disease so far as it is the cause of death.*[51]

Dr. Christian then discussed the aspects of influenza needing investigation. The first need was to find the cause of the disease, in particular the role of the influenza bacillus. Also, why was it that many people were only carriers of bacteria? Perhaps, Dr. Christian thought, a non-filterable organism might be worked out by human experimentation. Then there were the questions of protective vaccination and complicating organisms causing the pneumonias. As for treatment, he concluded, nothing seemed to be in any way effective.[52]

Next to speak at the meeting was Lieutenant Commander J.R. Phelps, representing the U.S. Navy's Medical Department. He, too, thought a "higher and higher percentage of cases" were being diagnosed as pneumonia. In several places, he noted, "it has been observed that there is a similarity of symptoms with the Bubonic Plague. The lungs do not look like the camp lungs of last year or certainly not the pneumonias the Rockefeller Institute is working on."[53] Perhaps the influenza bacillus was working symbiotically with another organism to cause the pneumonias. Some of the organisms that were being cultured from the lungs were much more pleomorphic (that is, variable in shape) than those in tuberculosis sputum, measles, etc.[54] Lieutenant Commander Phelps then asked: "Is not the plague bacillus in epidemics much more pleomorphic than [in] any ordinary circumstances? It seems there is an analogy between the Pfeiffer bacillus and plague bacillus."[55] In response, Dr. Joseph Goldberger of the U.S. Public Health Service's Hygienic Laboratory said: "We have had some cultures in the laboratory where the media gives a picture very much like plague bacillus."[56] Yet Dr. Goldberger thought the two diseases bore no relation.

Before the Commission adjourned, the members discussed: the difficulty of diagnosis at the patient's bedside; the question of immunity, particularly among those over thirty-five or forty; the way to prevent airborne infections; and how the work of the Commission could help physicians in the community.[57]

Much of the discussion during the later meetings of the Commission concerned the gathering of statistical epidemiological data, the great variation in the organisms causing the pneumonias, the problems relating to the production of safe and effective vaccines, and the failure of the experiments to produce influenza in Army and Navy volunteers. Lieutenant Commander Phelps concluded on December 20, 1918: "It does seem that we are justified in not pushing any form of mask or any form of vaccine, and to concentrate on one thing—ventilation. Plague comes where ventilation is not good....That is the only sanitary feature which stands out in the epidemic."[58] By mid-February of 1919, the Commission knew little more about the etiologic agent of influenza or how to treat the disease that it had in October.

During that same month, Dr. Rufus Cole of the Rockefeller Institute told Commission members that the random cultures taken at the Institute revealed that approximately thirty percent of the population normally harbored the influenza bacillus. Yet his group of respiratory investigators were still finding the bacillus in all cases clinically resembling influenza. He concluded:

> *One great difficulty is for us to find what influenza is and how to make the diagnosis. We are having in New York a great many acute respiratory diseases with fever. We have been going over all case histories during this epidemic and it is almost as difficult to see which was influenza—a very complex picture.*[59]

In the months following the Armistice, as medical professionals returned to their positions at the Rockefeller Institute, the Battle of the Flu had begun in earnest. According to Dr. George E. Vincent, Director of the Rockefeller Foundation, his organization would spend millions for medical research in 1919, particularly in the field of public health.[60] When Captain Francis G. Blake, of the Army's Pneumonia Commission, went on a week's leave to New York City at Christmas-time reporting to the Commandant of the Army Medical School at Washington, D.C., he found the whole Rockefeller crowd "working tooth and nail on this influenza business with monkeys and everything else...."[61] Back at his desk, the weary Captain wrote on January 2, 1919: "I shall be so glad when we get all this business off our hands and finished up and I can turn to something else for a change, as it seems as though I had done nothing but work on, and eat, and dream about, and live with pneumonia and influenza for six months."[62] But the reality was that he and many other medical scientists were just beginning the fight against respiratory disease. Blake and others continued to probe the influenza riddle throughout 1919.

At the same time, various government departments decided to sponsor a cooperative study of the statistics of the pandemic. In

January of 1919 the Surgeons General of the U.S. Army, U.S. Navy, and U.S. Public Health Service, and the Director of the Census designated the following men to form a joint influenza committee:

Bureau of the Census: Dr. William H. Davis (chairman) and Mr. C. S. Sloane

U.S. Public Health Service: Dr. Wade H. Frost and Mr. Edgar Sydenstricker

U.S. Navy: Lieutenant Commander J. R. Phelps and Surgeon Carroll Fox

U.S. Army: Colonel D. C. Howard, Colonel F. F. Russell and Lieutenant Colonel A. G. Love[63]

As early as December 1918, preliminary statistics of the pandemic had been reported to the section on vital statistics of the American Public Health Association during its meeting in Chicago. Then, in November the APHA had appointed its own Committee on Statistical Study of the Influenza Epidemic, chaired by Edwin W. Kopf of Metropolitan Life.[64] As a result of those efforts, within a few months statistical reports regarding influenza occurrences and mortality began to appear in print in a number of scientific and medical publications.

To Public Health Service statisticians Frost and Sydenstricker, early mortality statistical data were disappointing in that they could neither measure accurately the relative case incidence nor bring out important epidemiological data. Consequently, the two men set up a mechanism for special surveys in eighteen representative communities. What began as a statistical laboratory to investigate influenza later became a permanent Statistical Office in the Public Health Service under Sydenstricker's direction. In time a comprehensive history of influenza covering the years 1910 to 1935 would be produced by that office.[65] In addition, in the fall of 1919, Dr. Frost became Resident Lecturer at the new school of Hygiene and Public Health, then under the directorship of Dr. William H.

Welch, at Johns Hopkins University. Another person lured to the new Baltimore facility's staff was biostatistician Dr. Raymond Pearl.

While the gathering of statistics surged ahead, the research on protective vaccines for influenza and pneumonia proved disappointing. Shortly after the autumn wave of the pandemic began in 1918, newspapers reported that the Army Medical College was optimistic that the pnuemococcal vaccine it had tested during the summer months would effectively prevent pneumonia from complicating cases of influenza in the then-current epidemic and that there would soon be enough serum manufactured to vaccinate fifty thousand persons a day.[66] Then, in early October, the New York City Health Department announced that it had prepared and was testing a vaccine *directly* against influenza that utilized influenza bacilli. Although the new vaccine might be considered revolutionary by the public, the Health Commissioner said it was merely the result of applying "an old idea to a new disease."[67]

Laboratories in other major American cities also produced new vaccines, sometimes combining different bacterial species into one polyvalent serum. Alas, none seemed to prevent influenza. In fact, some of the vaccines, unfortunately, did more harm than good. For example, the *New York Times* reported on March 31, 1919, that 1,200 policemen in the city had reported sick after their serum injections. Police Captain John Ward of the East 35th St. Station and about ten of his patrolmen were reported to be badly disabled. Captain Ward was suffering from a swollen left arm, causing him to be confined to his home for two weeks.[68]

In Boston another type of serum injection became a popular antidote. Instead of a serum made from killed bacteria, the Boston Health Department decided to treat influenza-pneumonia patients with blood serum taken from influenza victims who had recovered from the disease. Consequently, in December the City Health Commissioner issued an appeal for former influenza sufferers to come forth and donate their blood to aid other flu victims.[69]

Boston's experimental serum did not provide the answer. At the American Medical Association's Convention in June, physicians were told that the influenza germ was still elusive. Dr. Wade Frost informed the doctors in attendance that the influenza investigators "had made little progress in isolating an organism of the disease or developing an antitoxin." And that—while sporadic outbreaks of influenza were anticipated in various communities—physicians would have to use their old methods of fighting the disease.[70]

The summer of 1919 was free of epidemic influenza. With the exception of occasional deaths from pneumonia—such as those of the Suffragist leader, Dr. Anna H. Shaw, on July 2 from a recurrence of pneumonia and Andrew Carnegie on August 11 at his Shadow Brook estate in Lenox, Massachusetts, of bronchial pneumonia—the nation's death rate was below normal during that summer. Many people credited the rainy weather with having depressed the usual seasonal fatalities.[71] But the rain did not cool the tempers of the thousands of unemployed and discontented across the country. People forgot about influenza for a while as they read about race riots in Washington, D.C. The war in Europe was over, but the soldiers were busy once again, on the American side of the ocean. Within a week of the trouble in Washington, other race riots in Chicago brought the National Guard into the streets of that city. Then, a few weeks later, guardsmen with machine guns faced mobs in Boston, as the police there went out on strike.

Riots, strikes, and the cost of living visibly increased as autumn neared, as did the fear of another deadly epidemic of influenza. In mid-August, New York City Health Commissioner Copeland warned people to guard their health carefully. He suggested that those who were weak should try to build up their strength to meet a possible recurrence of the flu. The Commissioner noted that the Health Department had received "anxious letters of inquiry from many parts of the country regarding the reappearance of the disease."[72] While uncertainty existed, he said, as to which age group would be attacked this time, he tended to believe there would be fewer fatalities. After all, those who had had the disease would practically be immune this time.[73]

Also preparing for another wave of illness was the National Red Cross. In late August it announced a campaign to raise fifteen million dollars, most of which would be used for the promotion of public health. The Red Cross also planned to increase its nursing services and broaden the Home Service divisions across the nation.[74]

In mid-September, Surgeon General Blue responded to the oft-repeated question: Will the flu come back this year? It was his opinion that it probably would. The Public Health Service now believed that the deadly wave of influenza in the fall of 1918 had not been a "fresh importation from abroad." A careful study of mortality statistics had revealed that there had been a "number of extensive though mild forerunners during the previous three or four years."[75] While the question of how much immunity a previous attack conferred was a mystery, one thing was certain: influenza was a communicable disease, spread not only by the sick but also by those "entirely well." Surgeon General Blue concluded:

> Communities should make plans now for dealing with any recurrences. The most promising way to deal with a possible recurrence is, to sum it up in a single word, _preparedness_. And now is the time to prepare.[76]

As the nation prepared for a new onslaught of disease, noted bacteriologists met in New York City in September to unite in an effort to find the etiologic agent of influenza. The four prominent medical scientists who sat in conference were: Dr. E.O. Jordan, professor of bacteriology at the University of Chicago; Dr. George W. McCoy, Director of the Hygienic Laboratory of the U.S. Public Health Service; Dr. William H. Park, Director of Laboratories of the New York City Department of Health; and Dr. M.J. Rosenau, Professor of Hygiene and Preventative Medicine at Harvard University. The conference, newspapers noted, marked the beginning of a federal, state, and municipal effort to prevent the threatened recurrent epidemic of influenza.[77]

New York City Health Commissioner Copeland announced at the same time that his department had a vaccine for those who wished to have an injection. The schools were making a rigorous daily inspection of all pupils, the teachers having been instructed in how to recognize the symptoms of influenza. In addition, the Health Department was planning to distribute a circular that would emphasize the importance of giving strict attention to any colds that might develop. It urged readers to isolate family members from the rest of the family, to sterilize their eating utensils and to make sure that the sick not sleep in the same bed with the well.[78]

September 1919 came and went, however, without any evidence of a new epidemic of influenza. Instead, the number of strikes and riots increased. In Omaha, national guardsmen were called in after a mob lynched Will Brown, a forty-five-year-old Negro, and hanged the Mayor twice, leaving him in critical condition.[79] And the President was ill again, having suffered a "nervous breakdown" on his western tour to gain support for the League of Nations. A week after the breakdown, President Wilson had a grave stroke. Doctors called in to consult on the case found the President to be a very sick man.[80]

Shortly thereafter, another Peace Conference veteran became ill again. On October 12, the *New York Times* noted that Colonel E. M. House was returning to the States suffering from a return of his "old malady." Although the newspaper reported that the old malady was probably influenza, the Colonel's physician, Dr. Albert Lamb, revealed a few days later that his patient's problem was another attack of renal colic.[81]

If influenza occurred only in scattered cases during the fall of 1919, more cases of "sleeping sickness" seemed to be turning up. The *Times* reported at the end of October that twenty-nine-year-old Mrs. Dora Mintz, from the Bronx, had been in one of the city's hospitals for two weeks in a comatose condition. Dr. Copeland said:

> *...she became ill October 1 with a sore throat which bothered her three days. On October 3 she felt better and attended a wedding. The next day she had a severe headache, and the following day she went to bed. She has been in a comatose condition since then.*
>
> *She was taken to the hospital October 16. She is receiving liquid nourishment, and it is said that at times she is delirious. The disease is comparatively rare. Some physicians believe it is an after-effect of influenza.*[82]

Mid-November found influenza cases now occurring among the scab workers who had been living for eight weeks in the strike-bound steel mills of Youngstown, Ohio.[83] But, thankfully, scattered cases remained the rule across the country. One flu victim in November was U.S. Senator Boies Penrose of Pennsylvania, who had collapsed from overwork following his part in the attempt to defeat the Versailles Treaty in the Senate. He was reported to be suffering from the grip, with his heart affected by the "almost incessant coughing to which he has been subjected for a few weeks."[84]

As the epidemic influenza remained away for the rest of 1919, health authorities began to believe that the pandemic pattern observed in 1891 might not recur. Perhaps deadly influenza was a thing of the past, after all. Perhaps.

7

A Tired Nation (1920)

The dinner of the National Efficiency Society which was to have been held last night at the Aldine Club, was postponed indefinitely on account of the epidemic of influenza.[1]

Nineteen twenty began quietly—and soberly. Although Prohibition did not go into effect for a few more weeks, many were afraid to risk drinking the alcoholic beverages that were available at their local bistros because, each week, scores of Americans were dying from spirits tainted with wood alcohol. On New Year's Eve, Broadway and Times Square lacked the usual pre-war Mardi Gras aura, with crowds of revelers carrying on till dawn. Nevertheless, many citizens were grateful that the old year had finally terminated. Unemployment, the high cost of living, riots and strikes, prolonged illnesses and the death of loved ones had made 1919 an unpleasant memory. The *New York Times* observed on January 1, 1920: "There were times during 1919 when the era leading up to the war seemed, in the casual retrospect, like some far-off golden age."[2] The American people hoped 1920 would bring happier and healthier times.

As the new year began, occasional reports of influenza epidemics recurring in far-removed areas of the world appeared in the newspapers. Influenza had reappeared in Spain, Japan and in the port of Rio de Janeiro. Soon came a report that hundreds of flu victims were dying daily in Poland.[3] Yet in the United States the news was good. On January 3 the Public Health Service announced that fewer than seven thousand cases of influenza had occurred since September 1. The greatest number had been reported in October, when 3,117 victims had been distributed over twenty-one states. Since October the number of cases reported had gradually declined. A Public Health Service official concluded: "It is too early to say that the danger point has passed, but it would seem safe to say that even should the epidemic recur within the next few months it would probably not be attended with so much pneumonia."[4]

Within a fortnight of that report, however, epidemic influenza reappeared across the nation, along with an increase in other respiratory diseases. The Assistant Secretary of the Navy, Franklin Delano Roosevelt, who was scheduled to speak to the Brooklyn Chamber of Commerce at a luncheon on January 10, had to postpone his appearance before the group because of a "severe cold."[5] New York City Health Commissioner Copeland was alarmed, on January 13, by the unusual increase in the number of measles cases reported in the City. In the previous ten days 2,221 cases had come to light, a remarkable number considering that only 8,194 cases had occurred in all of 1919. On the other hand, in 1918 there had been 28,075 cases of measles, with 790 deaths. Perhaps Dr. Copeland feared that the rising number of measles cases in early 1920 might be accompanied by increased respiratory infections of all kinds, as had occurred in 1918.[6]

At the same time that the Assistant Secretary of the Navy became ill, Johns Hopkins' Dr. Raymond Pearl started a prolonged bout with respiratory disease. On January 9 he went home from the office at noon, with a cold "palpably coming on." The following day he had the cold, and worked only until lunchtime, when he went home to nurse himself. Although he felt somewhat better the next day, he recorded in his diary on the eleventh that "Chases came in [the] afternoon and I got a flu germ from him."[7]

The hard-working Dr. Pearl went into the office the next day, but complained that his lungs were very bad. Home at noon again he went. On January 13 and the ensuing days, he made the following notations in his diary:

> *January 13 – Lungs warm. Called in Englehart. Very sick.*
> *January 14 – Very sick. Got nurse. Had influenza*
>   *bronchopneumonia. Darned near died.*
> *January 15 – Sick.*
> *January 16 – Out of danger.*
> *January 17 – In bed.*
> *January 18 – In bed.*
> *January 19 – Began to sit up in bed. Nurse left this afternoon.*
> *January 20 – Got up in chair in room.*
> *January 21 – Dressed and downstairs. Reed came out in P.M.*
>   *about a lab matter. Proof came from Jawle.*[8]

Although Dr. Pearl felt first rate on January 22, his chipper mood was short-lived. Not only was he weak and feeble for the next few days, but his entire family in turn had fallen ill. His young daughter, he reported, who was running a high temperature, was obviously sick, and his wife was in bad shape. On January 25, he commented: "Altogether family in low state." Two days later Pearl went into the office for the first time since the onset of his illness, but on the thirtieth he was still rather tired and worn out.[9]

What was happening in the Pearl household in Baltimore was occurring in other homes all across the country. For example, sickness had reinvaded the Robert Frost homestead in Amherst, Massachusetts. On January 28 the poet wrote to his daughter Lesley in New York that "Mama's been taking care of sick children till she's had to give up sick herself." He added:

I've been wanting to say the word, come home for your free week; but I don't know that you wouldn't be better off where you are. You've got an infirmary to go to if you are sick (you needn't think I'm asking you to be sick) and you haven't any responsibility for sick people. By staying, too, you avoid two train journeys more or less risky the way things are. What do you say?[10]

On January 15, health officers in Chicago suddenly stirred into increased activity when doctors reported five hundred cases of influenza and pneumonia, with twenty deaths. City Health Commissioner John Dill Robertson thereupon announced that he would organize the three thousand graduate nurses in the area into squads, to ensure that nurses would be available in every part of the city. As soon as a case of influenza developed, the victim's house would be tagged. Commissioner Robertson strongly urged Chicago citizens to wage a defensive campaign against a possible recurrence of epidemic influenza.[11]

On that same day Washington, D.C. seemed to be less affected by flu than the Windy City. Capital area physicians reported only twenty-one cases of the disease on January 15, but it was the largest number reported on any one day since the previous October. Within a few days, however, influenza once again became a killer in the district. On January 20, there were eighty-six flu victims with two deaths. But Health Officer Fowler suspected that many people were probably suffering only from "colds," or "grip," rather than the flu. Two days later the daily total of new flu cases reached 226. Still the local health authorities continued to insist that the influenza was not an epidemic. By the twenty-third such optimism was hardly warranted, however, as the *Washington Post* reported the absence of twenty thousand pupils and eighty teachers. The "already war-worn" school system of the district, the paper noted, was in chaos as in the fall of 1918.[12]

Once again, trained nurses were in short supply. One result was a sudden surge of women enrolling in Red Cross classes for home hygiene and instruction in the home care of the sick. On January 27, when twenty states reported influenza was on the increase, the United States Senate passed a $500,000 Influenza Appropriation for research purposes, although as originally introduced the resolution had called for $5,000,000. Congressional hearts that had remained cool to the appeals for research funds all through 1919 suddenly warmed somewhat, as their own families became influenza victims.[13]

Even before the senators offered to open up their pockets, a movement was underway in the House to amend the *Volstead Act*, making alcoholic stimulants more easily obtainable for the duration of the epidemic. On January 23 an Illinois Representative submitted a proposal to relax for ninety days restrictions on stimulants obtained by doctors' prescriptions. The "wet measure" would make it possible for reputable physicians to prescribe such quantities of whiskey as they believed necessary, without having to obey the current limitation of one pint or less per patient every ten days.[14] Encouraging such changes in the Prohibition legislation was the New York County Medical Society. On January 30, its officers wrote to the Surgeon General of the Public Health Service to urge that federal authorities supply, at conveniently situated depots, alcoholic stimulants for the care of the sick, and guarantee the purity and nature of the stimulants to be so dispensed. They reminded the Surgeon General:

> *The great majority of the people believe that alcoholic beverages as a stimulant and food are often a necessity and they demand the same, and in this they are supported by the medical profession. Under the present conditions some are fortunate in having a supply of stimulants, while it is absolutely impossible for others to obtain any. Those who may be licensed to dispense liquor cannot guarantee its purity.*[15]

Of course, the Public Health Service lacked authority to set up liquor depots. And the "drys" were still too powerful to permit any changes in the Prohibition legislation. City health departments had to purchase and distribute their own alcoholic supplies.

While Congress considered legislation to combat the epidemic, the ranks of the District's police and fire departments grew thinner as influenza claimed one man after another. On January 28, more than three hundred school teachers were out sick. By that date officials of the various government departments estimated that at least one-fifth of their employees were ailing.[16] Within another week the numbers affected rose even higher. On February 5 Secretary of the Interior Franklin K. Lane wrote to a friend: "All my force is sick ...680 in my Department are in bed."[17] While Lane himself evidently escaped the virus, other Cabinet members did not. On January 27 the *Washington Post* revealed that three cabinet officials, Secretary of State Lansing, Secretary of War Baker, and Attorney General A. Mitchell Palmer, were all home with "colds."

Another Washingtonian to become sick with flu at this time was Wisconsin's Senator Robert M. LaFollette. Already ailing with an intermittent pain in his side when Congress reconvened in January, the Senator, who was unable to attend the opening sessions, decided he had better go to the Mayo Clinic in Rochester, Minnesota, for a medical examination. Because of a bout with influenza and an infected tooth, however, he did not leave for the clinic until January 20. There, after a thorough check extending over a period of seventeen days, Drs. Will and Charles Mayo decided the Senator needed to have his gallbladder removed. But not just then. Except for emergency procedures, surgery at the clinic was unwise while the influenza epidemic prevailed. In consequence, the Mayos suggested to LaFollette that he return to Madison and keep a minimum schedule of activities until conditions in Rochester were more favorable for surgery. The Senator finally had his operation on June 7.[18]

The Wisconsin Republican Senator's own health problems were the culmination of a series of medical crises in his family extending over a period of two years. In January 1918 his son Bob, Jr., who had been working in Washington, D.C., had developed streptococcal pneumonia. The young LaFollette was gravely ill for many months, sometimes appearing to be improving, but then relapsing into acute periods of intense pain. In July 1918 he was finally well enough to be moved to Hot Springs, Virginia. After Hot Springs came a year's convalescence in California. For the Senator, his son's illness brought on worry and bills: bills from doctors, nurses, and hospitals; bills that consumed his salary month after month— and separation from his wife, who remained with her ailing son in California for nearly a year. Recuperation from pneumonia could be a lengthy and costly process.[19]

On January 29, 1920, just as a new relief hospital for flu victims opened up in Washington, Health Officer Fowler announced that the epidemic had probably peaked in the district. He was right. The number of deaths from influenza and pneumonia in Washington for the week ending on the tenth of January had been 22; on the seventeenth, 27; on the twenty-fourth, 81; and, on the thirty-first, 181. The following week, February 7, there were 164, and the decline continued in the ensuing weeks.[20]

One of the influenza fatalities during the week ending January 31 in the district was the grand-nephew of George Washington, Laurence Washington, born at Mount Vernon in 1855. For many years he had been in charge of the Congressional Reading Room at the Library of Congress; he died on the twenty-eighth, having been ill for only a week.[21]

A more prominent Washington personality to succumb to influenza at the end of January was Senator John Bankhead of Alabama, who, at the age of seventy-seven, was the oldest member of the upper house. Although at first his medical condition did not appear to be serious, death came on March 1. Senator Bankhead had been a long-time Washington area resident, first as a U.S.

Congressman for eighteen years beginning in 1887, and then as a member of the Senate. He had been the sole-surviving member to have served in the Confederate Army.[22]

More fortunate than Senator Bankhead in his battle with the flu was Senator Hiram Johnson of California, whose bout in early February occurred just as he returned from a strenuous speaking tour in the midwest. The California Progressive Republican, who had presidential aspirations in 1920, returned to his Senate seat in ten days, still tired, but apparently recovered from the flu.[23]

Or was it the flu? A famous Ottawa physician, the *Washington Post* noted on January 29, was insisting that the present epidemic raging in North America was not influenza. Indeed, according to Dr. H. C. Church, "there will be no recurrence of the influenza epidemic in this generation." The cases that were being reported daily in the New York and Chicago newspapers were "nothing more or less than grip." The present symptoms, the doctor said, were "no different and the death rate no higher than of the old and more familiar affliction." None of his own patients who had fallen ill in the deadly 1918 wave seemed to be affected this time. Dr. Church believed that those who had been ill in 1918 had been immunized against the current infecting agent, while those who had not been attacked in 1918 were not susceptible to the disease at all: "This scourge undoubtedly has swept the world in past ages....But a generation, or perhaps many generations, will elapse before it comes again in the deadly form that it did in 1918."[24]

Still, confusion continued to exist in the relationship between "grip," "influenza," and pneumonia. Some physicians labeled their seriously-ill patients as flu victims; other doctors used the term pneumonia. Meanwhile, the U. S. Public Health Service finally announced on January 31 that influenza was epidemic throughout the country. The disease, the service believed, was evidently uninfluenced by the weather since it was just as prevalent in the southern states as elsewhere.[25]

But the course of the disease in 1920 was as erratic as it had been in the fall of 1918. Some communities had high morbidity and mortality rates; others were only moderately affected. New York City suffered severely in 1920. Indeed, more cases of influenza were reported in a single day in New York City in early 1920 than on any day during the autumn wave of the disease in 1918. However, nationwide the 1920 epidemic lasted for only twelve weeks instead of thirty-one as in 1918-19. As a result, far fewer deaths occurred in 1920. There were enough, nonetheless, to make it the second deadliest influenza epidemic to appear thus far in the twentieth century. Within eight weeks' time in early 1920, more than eleven thousand people died from influenza and/or pneumonia in just two cities, Chicago and New York. Statistics gathered in later years showed that the excess mortality rate (per 100,000) during the 1918-19 epidemic had been 550.5, while the rate in early 1920 was 97.2.[26]

New York City's Health Commissioner Copeland had repeatedly congratulated the residents of his city throughout 1919 for having had one of the lower mortality rates among the larger cities in the fall of 1918. He believed the lower mortality rate had been the result of a cautious citizenry and the realistic preventive policies that the city had adopted during the pandemic. Whereas Washington, D.C., had closed its schools in 1918, those in New York City had remained open. They would remain so in 1920. Commissioner Copeland was adamant in his decision to keep the schools running:

If every school teacher in the city were taken ill I would hire entertainers to keep the public schools open. We have a million children in the schools, and every minute they are in school their parents know where they are and that they are under supervision. Of the school children, probably 700,000 come from tenement homes. We know what those homes are and how sometimes several persons are crowded into two small rooms. Such children

are better off in school. . . . There they are inspected by the teachers.
If a child gives evidence of having a cold or feels ill, that child is
separated from the others and examined by a doctor. If it is found
that the child has influenza, he is sent home, under the care of
the Board of Health, and the Board of Health decides whether
home conditions are good or whether the child must be sent to a
hospital.[27]

As influenza once again neared the epidemic stage in New York City, the city fathers quickly voted an emergency $80,000 appropriation to provide for sufficient nurses and home inspectors, and for the medical supplies that would be required in the Battle of the Flu. But as thousands of New Yorkers fell sick, the available supply of nurses was simply inadequate. Commissioner Copeland then sent out an appeal throughout the East for "practical nurses" who would be paid at a rate of $4.00 a day, and for "household workers" who would receive $3.50.[28]

As if sickness were not enough, food supplies in the cities grew less plentiful as the winter of 1920 wore on. The reason, said Director General of Railroads Walker D. Hines, was that influenza had seriously affected railway freight traffic. "Coupled with bad weather conditions," said the railroad administrator, "the influenza epidemic has dealt a serious blow to railroad operation." Scores of railroad workers were now ill, nursing dangerously ill members of their families, or dealing with the funerals of loved ones.[29]

As in 1918, the law of supply and demand increased the cost of much-needed supplies during the epidemic. One group who made out well were those druggists who dispensed alcoholic beverages for "medicinal purposes." At a time when the New York City Health Department was buying eight hundred gallons of whiskey at ten to eleven dollars a gallon, some retail druggists were selling half-pints for as much as seven dollars.[30]

Once again, the price of coffins suddenly went up. The National Casket Company announced on January 29 that due to a "sharp rise in the price of lumber of all grades," and the high cost and shortage of the textiles used to line the caskets, the price list in circulation would change immediately. The announcement outraged Commissioner Copeland, who threatened to seek a federal investigation.[31]

Influenza also raised the price of many household items, including that of lemons by fifty percent. Lemons which had sold for twenty cents a dozen in mid-January were thirty cents at the beginning of February. New York housewives were irate. Grocers blamed the flu epidemic:

> 'You see,' said one grocer yesterday, 'when a person begins to feel a cold coming, he immediately thinks he is going the have the flu. The first thing he does is to buy lemons with which to make a hot lemonade before going to bed. The demand for lemons was doubled at the start of the influenza epidemic, and at present it has quadrupled. The result has been a scarcity of lemons in the market, and naturally the law of supply and demand had to have its effect. That's why the price of lemons has advanced fifty percent.'[32]

Such profiteering during and after the pandemic called forth some federal action from the Justice Department. Armin W. Riley, Special Assistant to Attorney General Palmer, became the head of a flying squadron, organized to arrest and issue indictments against greedy businessmen. By early August 1920, the Justice Department had made 1,854 arrests, with 1,499 indictments returned and 151 convictions.[33]

In the meantime, February found influenza still increasing in many states. The New York State Legislature quickly responded to an appeal from its chief executive, Governor Alfred E. Smith, by voting an appropriation of $50,000 to fight the epidemic. Both the Governor and Mrs. Smith were sick in bed. According to the *Washington Post*, the Albany executive mansion had virtually become a hospital. The Empire State legislature also reconsidered, at that time, the need to pass a "health risk" bill that would provide New York State residents with compulsory health risk insurance. The resolution had little chance of success, however, with labor leader Samuel Gompers turning up in Albany to work against its passage. According to Gompers, compulsory health insurance would only add to the power over the people. American labor in 1920 feared "big government." Elsewhere in the country, Minnesota Governor J. A. A. Burnquist's influenza had turned into pneumonia. The epidemic appeared to be waning in Massachusetts, but was on the increase in Kansas. In the nation as a whole, the 1920 epidemic apparently crested during the second week in February.[34]

Early in February, the President's physician, Dr. Grayson, revealed that his patient, now invalided since October, had contracted a cold several days before, and had had a narrow escape from influenza. Happily, the president was "steadily, though slowly, improving" from his stroke, and was now walking about the second floor of the White House unassisted.[35]

It was already apparent by February 3 that the Ottawa physician's contention that those who had been victims in 1918 were this time immune was mere optimism. Too many people fell sick again in 1920 for that to be true. Indeed, Dr. Hans Zinsser believed he had suffered three attacks of influenza during the pandemic, the last siege being the most serious because of a complicating pneumonia.[36]

Speculation as to the cause of influenza continued. In Paris the more elderly members of society tended to blame the increased mortality among young females on the shocking new styles of clothing worn by the French younger set. Nonsense, declared a Paris medical expert. Low bodices and short skirts did not bring on influenza: mademoiselle "may catch influenza through her nose, but never through her limbs or shoulders."[37]

On the American side of the Atlantic, the *Denver Post*

announced on February 3 that it would give $25,000 to any physician who could find a cure for influenza. The money would be awarded after the Rockefeller Foundation and the Johns Hopkins University had approved the proposed cure.[38] But during the 1920 crisis most physicians were too busy tending to the sick to give much time to devising new cures. Some doctors even found themselves back in the U.S. Army. Since the first week of February, Surgeon General Ireland recalled one hundred officers in the Medical Reserve Corps back to active service to help combat flu.[39]

The Army had found its ranks being rapidly depleted by influenza once again. However, in 1920 the problem was confined to one side of the Atlantic. With the exception of the American occupation troops who would remain on the Rhine, the demobilization process was drawing to a close. The last contingent of U.S. troops to leave Brest had sailed in mid-January on the U.S.S. *George Washington*. General Pershing was now back in the United States, making a country-wide inspection tour of the camps. The general, a flu victim in 1918, fell sick with flu once again, this time at Forth Worth, Texas. Fortunately, his case was a slight one.[40]

The General was lucky that he was situated in Texas when he came down with the flu during that second week of February. Citizens in the village of Cummington, in the Hampshire hills west of Northampton, Massachusetts, were struck by a blizzard as well as influenza that week. All roads to the tiny village were cut off for days, and the community's supplies of food and medicine rapidly dwindled. The two overworked physicians tending to the sick in the village had to telephone the Northampton Red Cross for aid in breaking through the snow-choked roads so that much-needed supplies could be brought in.[41]

American Indians also suffered severely from epidemic influenza in the early months of 1920, much as they had in the previous deadly wave of the disease. In one small Piute village in Inyo County, California, the rural mail carrier found every inhabitant stricken with the disease in the latter part of February. None in the village had received medical attention, and more than one hundred victims died that month.[42]

As the influenza epidemic progressed, the director of the State Department of Public Health in Springfield, Illinois, became concerned with the increased number of cases of "sleeping sickness" (lethargic encephalitis) being reported to his agency. During the week ending February 9, there were sixteen new cases, many occurring in post-influenzal patients.[43] The same disease seemed to be cropping up in greater numbers in New York City. On February 27, a twenty-seven-year-old intern at the Lincoln Hospital in the Bronx died of sleeping sickness after lying in a coma for several hours. The doctor had been attending two other victims of the strange disease, one of whom had died. On March 9 the *New York Times* quoted Dr. Copeland as saying that there were more cases of lethargic encephalitis than ever before. Since January 1 the City Health Department had recorded 175 cases, with 40 deaths.[44]

March began with frigid temperatures plaguing much of the country. The northeast had to dig itself out from another blizzard as the month wore on. Such bitter, raw weather did little to help the influenza sufferers and although the epidemic had reached its peak, new cases continued to erupt in many of the nation's communities. On the day in early March when Senator Bankhead's death was reported, the announcement came that one of the nation's foremost writers, William Dean Howells, age eighty-three, was ill with influenza in Savannah, Georgia, and was passing his birthday in bed.[45] Another March victim was Secretary of Labor William B. Wilson, who, because of his illness, was unable to attend the Seventh Anniversary Dinner of the Department of Labor on the fourth. The Secretary had been scheduled to be the guest of honor at the affair.[46]

Not feeling much better as March began was Dr. Pearl. By that time he was thoroughly immersed in "flu work," the statistical studies instituted by the Frost-Sydenstricker group in Washington. Baltimore had suffered from bad weather and widespread sickness in February, and on February 15 Dr. Pearl had again recorded in his diary that he had a raw throat and was not feeling well. It was the onset of another forced retirement to his bed. Not until February 25 was he able to return to the laboratory for a half-day's work. Even then, he was still unwell. Two days later he described himself as feeling wretched; the weather was miserable, and he thought he had another cold coming on. Perhaps he'd better see a doctor soon. For the time being, however, he continued to work, but only for half-days, in the hope that a reduced work schedule and longer rest periods might restore his health. Yet as March progressed, the statistician came down with another cold; at which time he did seek medical help. After a thorough examination, his doctor advised him that his lungs were in bad shape, and that he must take a rest. As a result, Pearl made arrangements to head for a warmer clime. On March 31, Dr. and Mrs. Pearl sailed from Baltimore to recuperate in the Carolinas. When they returned in mid-April Pearl was feeling somewhat better, but his wife had taken sick on the trip and was still "pretty weak."[47]

Pearl's health problems had begun early in January and even as late as May, he was still complaining of feeling tired. A similar lethargy existed among those who had been flu victims in early 1920 in the Robert Frost household. The Frosts had gone north to their farm in Franconia, New Hampshire, when Amherst College closed at the end of the first semester. The poet had decided, apparently rather suddenly, to leave his teaching post at the college for a life of farming and writing. Then the storm that struck Cummington, Massachusetts, rolled over Franconia as well. On February 8, Frost wrote to Lesley, at Barnard College, that they were snowed in by "the greatest snow-storm of all time ....We are running short of food, fuel and water.... Everybody is frightened but Marjorie.... who doesn't know enough....to appreciate the seriousness of snow actually halfway up our windows."[48] In April Lesley finally received a letter from her mother, who had been unwell since January. Mrs. Frost began her letter with:

> *I am sorry I haven't written for so long. I don't know what is the matter with me. Most of the time I feel as if I <u>couldn't</u> write a letter. And it's pretty mean of me, too .... Papa wrote you about Jean. Since that happened I haven't been sleeping well....*
>
> *Marjorie hasn't been to school yet. After she had the grippe she didn't seem to get at all strong and the very day school began, she woke up with a fierce sick headache, and for two days vomited up all the medicine I gave her, and she couldn't eat a thing for about 4 days. I had to call Dr. Johnson. She is much better now but has grown rather thin, and is behind in her work.*[49]

"Jean" was Jean Frost, the younger, school-teacher sister of the poet. An arch-opponent of America's entry to World War I, she had, according to the poet, become "everything she could think of" during the war, to express her extreme antipathy to it: "Pro-German, pacifist, internationalist, draft obstructor, and seditionist." In the fall of 1918 she had turned up at Robert and Elinor's home in Amherst, a fugitive from a mob in Mill River, Massachusetts, that was threatening to throw her into a mill pond unless she kissed the flag. Jean's emotional behavior had become erratic and confused. Needless to say, she had much difficulty in landing and holding a teaching position when the townspeople discovered her political opinions.[50]

Jean Frost and a friend had spent the winter of 1919-20 in Lowell and Haverhill, Massachusetts. Both women had caught influenza, but apparently managed to take care of themselves. After that, Jean went to Portland, Maine. Towards the end of March Robert Frost learned that his sister was being confined by the Portland police, as a demented woman, still ranting and raving on the subject of war. As one would expect, Jean became the poet's constant concern as the spring progressed. His sister had moved about the New England states so often that it was difficult to decide which state would bear the responsibility to provide long-term custodial care if it became necessary. Frost himself lacked the financial means to put her in a private institution. He hoped that her "pronounced insanity" might be only a temporary condition. More than that, Frost felt that his sister's demented behavior was not entirely emotionally-based. He wrote to his friend, Louis Untermeyer:

> There remains only Jean to speak of. Why will she let the spirit be dragged down sick by the sick body? If the spirit were sick in its own right I shouldn't be preaching this sermon. But it is the body uttering its sickness through the spirit—I can tell by the sound. I suppose I should distrust any sickness of the spirit as from the body unless I knew for certain that the body had a clean bill of health from the medical dept. A sick spirit in a sound body for me.[51]

More than a few psychiatrists during the pandemic years believed that mental disorders sometimes followed influenza, especially among those who had histories of emotional problems. Whether Jean Frost's siege of influenza in 1920 triggered her severe breakdown in March is impossible to determine, but it was at least a possibility. In any event, the Frost family was constantly preoccupied with health matters, mental and physical, throughout the first half of 1920—and beyond. To make matters worse, the poet was ill again in September with jaundice.[52]

As March of 1920 progressed, influenza cases lessened across the country. This was the good news; the bad was that the already high cost of living was rising with each passing month. From January 1919 to January 1920 wholesale costs jumped an average of twenty-two percent. Clothes soared by more than forty-nine percent; food, twenty-two percent; household furnishings, more than forty-eight percent; fuel and lighting, eight percent; and metals three percent.[53] Meatpackers blamed consumers for the high prices of meat: Americans ate "too high up on the hog." Consequently, an example would be set in the White House. Mrs. Wilson planned to serve cheaper cuts, and to share her economical recipes with the nation's housewives.[54]

Because March was so frigid and blustery in the east, it was April before some ailing Washingtonians dared return to their posts. Arriving back at his Senate desk on April 1 after weeks of "laryngitis" was Pennsylvania's Philander C. Knox, who had been one of the irreconcilable opponents of the League of Nations. His reappearance in the Senate meant that the Keystone State had at least one of its two Senators in attendance, for Boies Penrose was still suffering from the bout with influenza and its complications that he had had in November 1919.[55]

April was less kind to Broadway star John Barrymore than to Senator Knox. In the latter part of January the idolized stage and screen actor had had a siege of flu, forcing him to drop out of the cast of *The Jest* for a few days. The rest period was too short. As the weeks went by, with Barrymore rehearsing a new play and shooting a movie at the same time, he grew progressively more tired and physically run-down. The opening of the play, *Richard III*, was postponed some five days to let its star get much-needed rest. Then, when the drama finally opened, mid-week matinees were cancelled to give the actor additional rest. Nonetheless, on April 3 the *New York Times* reported that John Barrymore had suffered a "nervous breakdown."[56]

A few days later, that newspaper's theatrical section described the nature of Barrymore's so-called breakdown in greater detail. After spending several hours with the ailing idol, the *Times* reporter declared that Mr. B.'s illness was hardly a breakdown, but simply an intense and immeasurable fatigue due to overwork. Barrymore had told him that he was not only unable to play Richard at that moment, but that he was "literally incapable of standing on his feet for the period of time which Richard required."[57] Like so many flu victims, Barrymore had the familiar wobbly legs. As a result, the actor announced that he would refuse roles and rest until the autumn.

Such a course of action was undoubtedly wise. On April 19 the *Times* noted the death of the daughter of former Supreme Court Justice and Presidential candidate Charles Evans Hughes, Miss Helen Hughes, twenty-eight, after a "long attack of influenza and pneumonia" dating to September of 1918. Her death was attributed to "advanced tuberculosis" following upon the heels of the earlier illnesses. Breakdowns—tubercular, mental, and physical—were all too common sequelae to influenza.[58]

The nationwide influenza epidemic of 1920 finally ended in April. Influenza, however, continued to interrupt people's schedules and, indeed, to claim lives as the year progressed. On May 12, newspapers announced that the author William Dean Howells had died suddenly, the day before, from the influenza he had caught in March. In the last week of May came news that Pennsylvania Senator Penrose had had a "relapse," and was suffering from fatigue occasioned by "prolonged conferences with political leaders."[59]

A week later, Senator Penrose, who was considered by some political observers as the boldest and most resourceful of the older Republican chiefs, announced that he was determined to go to the Republican Convention in Chicago in June "if it kills me." The arch-politician had a bevy of physicians in consultation over his health as June began. Finally, the doctors convinced Penrose that if he defied their advice to rest in his home he might never return to active politics. It was a bitter pill for Penrose to swallow, for he had been considered the logical leader for the presidential convention. Penrose had to settle for telephone communications with the other party bosses as they chose Ohio Senator Warren G. Harding for their standard-bearer.[60]

Another long-time Republican figure whose presence was missed at the Chicago convention was George W. Perkins, who in 1912 had managed Theodore Roosevelt's Progressive Party campaign in the three-way fight for the presidency won by Woodrow Wilson. On June 11, 1920, the news' services reported Perkins to be ill of a "nervous collapse," and residing in a private sanatorium in Stamford, Connecticut. His nervous collapse was the sequel to months and months of suffering from the "after-effects of influenza and pneumonia," which he had contracted in January of 1919 while in France.[61]

Perkins, who had lost his seven months' pregnant daughter-in-law, Katherine, to influenza in the fall of 1918, had been chairman of the Finance Committee of the Y.M.C.A. during the war. Sometime after the Armistice, he had gone to France to inspect the Y.M.C.A. facilities and visit his son, who was then serving with the U.S. Army of Occupation in Coblenz, Germany. In mid-January 1919 Perkins fell ill with broncho-pneumonia and was bedded down in the American Hospital in Paris. From that siege of illness, the former businessman-turned-civic-leader never recovered. For months he was confined to his home, under the care of his family physician in New York. Later, physicians in consultation decided that a sojourn in the Catskills might speed along his recuperation. As 1920 progressed, however, many of his old Progressive party associates tried to interest him in the coming Republican Convention and were urging him to make the effort to attend. To no avail. Perkins died June 18, in his fifty-eighth year, of "acute inflammation of the brain." The death certificate, the *New York Times* reported, gave the cause as "acute encephalitis," with a secondary cause being "chronic myocarditis." Perkins was one of those unfortunate individuals with a post-influenzal encephalitis.[62]

Another nationally-prominent Republican politician to succumb to the ever-increasing acute encephalitis, or what was still called in 1920 "sleeping sickness," was the heir to the paper manufacturing business in Dalton, Massachusetts, W. Murray Crane. The wealthy businessman had twice represented the Bay State in the United States Senate, and was a supporter of the man chosen to be the Republican Vice-Presidential candidate in 1920, Calvin Coolidge. He had gone to Chicago in June, hoping to win an endorsement for the League of Nations from his party, but returned home without accomplishing his purpose, and—according to the newspapers—with his health impaired. A few weeks later, while attending the Coolidge notification ceremonies, Crane collapsed with what the papers called heat exhaustion. However, his condition deteriorated with each passing week, and he was eventually confined to bed. After a four or five day sleep, the politician died on October 1, yet another victim of "inflammation of the brain," or acute encephalitis.[63]

Pennsylvania's Senator Penrose fared better in his long battle with the after-effects of the flu. On August 4 it was announced that the Senator had gone for an automobile ride on the previous day, the first time he had ventured forth from his home in three months. Penrose expected that he would be able to return to the Senate shortly thereafter. The announcement, unfortunately, was premature. It was not until January 3, 1921, that the Pennsylvanian was to appear again in the Senate, after a thirteen months illness.[64]

Republicans managed nicely without the services of their ailing Pennsylvania boss through the fall of 1920. In the Presidential election between Democrat James Cox and Republican Harding, the GOP won a landslide victory. The grumbling and rebellion among the American people that had begun in 1918 and continued through 1919 and 1920 were amply reflected in the votes tallied in the polling stations on November 2. For example, the Michigan township of Frankenmuth in Saginaw County, which for thirty years had gone Democratic by huge majorities, gave Harding 954 votes and Cox a mere 14.[65]

While many political analysts through the intervening years have suggested that the 1920 results were less an endorsement of Harding than a resounding anti-administration vote, one must give Harding credit for using the soothing language people wanted to hear: "America's present need is not heroics but healing; not nostrums but normalcy; not revolution but restoration.... not surgery but serenity."[66] How appropriate such words were at a time when the public was recuperating in a physical sense. Harding was criticized for his coining of the word "normalcy." Yet perhaps those who listened to him in 1920 were more influenced by the other words he used: healing, restoration, serenity. Good health and happiness were what most people hoped for.

Happily for the nation, epidemic influenza was scarcely evident as 1920 began its final month. At the same time, however, a new influenza-related malady made its appearance. Newspapers reported early in December that all of Paris was suffering from a curious and unusual epidemic of hiccoughs, apparently accompanying "influenza colds." The disease was evidently highly contagious, affecting one family member after another, including the family of President A. Millerand. The disease was so widespread that for the first time in history physicians were treating hiccoughs seriously. French medical authorities said that while it was not the first time hiccoughs were noticed accompanying influenza, never before had they been such a conspicuous feature.[67]

Before the year ended, the strange malady had traveled to the American side of the Atlantic. On December 19, Acting Secretary of State Norman H. Davis was prostrated by a hiccoughs attack in Washington, D.C. Then, a few days later, on December 23, the New York Times revealed that an epidemic of hiccoughs had erupted in New York City. Dr. Copeland was describing the disease as a "nervous form of influenza," with seizures lasting from twenty-four to forty hours. Fortunately, the new nervous ailment did not seem to be causing any fatalities.[68]

Yet the nation was saddened once more by the death in December of one of its new young heroes, Notre Dame's All-American football star George Gipp. The senior gridman had fallen ill with pneumonia following the Notre Dame–Northwestern game on November 20. According to the press releases, Chicago medical specialists had succeeded in ridding his system of pneumonia, but Gipp "did not have the stamina to ward off the poison resulting from the throat infection."[69] After a fourth relapse, he died on December 14. Notre Dame coaches immortalized the young man in later years with the dressing room plea: "Let's win one for the Gipper."

Nineteen twenty ended soberly, but less quietly than it had begun. On New Year's Eve, Broadway and Times Square looked more like the old days, although there was little raucous behavior. That evening former Secretary of the Interior F. K. Lane wrote to a friend: "It is the last night of an unhappy year."[70] The news from across the world had turned more dismal as month had followed month. By December China and Central Europe were in the grip of famines; race riots were occurring in Independence, Kansas; New York City was in the midst of a crime wave, as were Philadelphia, Baltimore, Cincinnati and Pittsburgh. Former soldiers, now jobless and disgruntled, were being blamed for the rampant robberies. And, more than seventy-five thousand men were idle in Detroit, for people were not buying automobiles.[71]

In a letter to Ray Stannard Baker, Kansas editor William Allen White described the conditions and the mood of the people as 1920 came to an end:

> What a God-damned world this is! I trust you will realize that I am not swearing; merely trying to express in the mildest terms what I think of the conditions that exist. What a God-damned world!
>
> Starvation on the one hand, and indifference on the other, pessimism rampant, faith quiescent, murder met with indifference, the lowered standard of civilization faced with universal complaisance, and the whole story so sad that nobody can tell it.
>
> If anyone had told me ten years ago that our country would be what it is today, and that the world would be what it is today, I should have questioned his reason.[72]

A story so sad that nobody could tell it. The world of 1920 had become so grief-stricken that it had been stunned into apathy and silence. It needed time to heal itself. Disease had been more deadly and crippling than all of the guns and gases of the years 1914-1918. Almost every family had personally been affected by the pestilence that had stridden across the world not once but repeatedly. The impact of disease on private lives had been extraordinary. In later years people would often say of the men who had been gassed during the war that they were "never the same again." But the same words also described so many of the victims of the pandemic. The pandemic simply changed people's lives: it made six-year-old Mary McCarthy and her brothers orphans; parents and familiar surroundings vanished almost overnight. It was a time of tears, and when the tears no longer fell, they oftentimes became internal tears.

Consequently, the world of 1920 was both a sad and sickly one. Frederick Lewis Allen wrote, a generation or more later, that people were tired in the three or four years that followed the Armistice: "their public spirit, their consciences, and their hopes were tired."[73] But their bodies were tired as well. It was literally a sick world that they were living in. John Dewey wrote early in 1923 that he doubted if the consciousness of sickness had ever been so widespread as it was then. There was a "pervasive and overhanging" awareness of disease.[74] The deadly pandemic waves of influenza had left a train of ailing victims with Bright's disease, cardiac irregularities, vascular problems, pulmonary tuberculosis, and a host of nervous and paralytic afflictions. It was truly a sick and tired nation—in a sick and tired world.

8

The Battle Continues

For the medical profession, the 1918 influenza pandemic was a humbling experience. The great strides made in bacteriology during the fifty years preceding the pandemic had given many scientists a false sense of security, particularly in their belief that the production of appropriate vaccines would prevent most communicable diseases from getting out of hand. But before vaccines could be made, the identity of the infecting agents had to be known. In 1918 medical science was unable to discover the cause of influenza.

While the pandemic may have perplexed and frustrated physicians, it kindled a vigorous crusade against disease in the United States and abroad. Institutions such as the Rockefeller Institute and Hospital spent hundreds of millions of dollars in the post-pandemic years to study respiratory diseases and to find the etiology of influenza. Within months of the cessation of World War I, medical professionals from around the globe met at Cannes, France to formulate plans for a permanent international Red Cross organization that would work for improved public health and disease eradication.

Indeed, the war years ushered in the era of the rise of public health consciousness with its special emphasis on preventive medicine. The influenza pandemic was a catastrophic event in human history, one that made people acutely aware of disease and of the need for its prevention.

This new consciousness of disease was a natural result of the pandemic because so many families had buried loved ones or had been forced to cope with long-term illnesses that apparently were the sequelae to influenza. Certain words—tottering, tired, emaciated—keep reappearing in the memoirs of those who were victims of the pandemic. People like John Barrymore and the actress, Eva Le Gallienne, were literally unable to stand on their feet for any extended length of time. Victims tired easily, and were often cross and out-of-sorts. Because the disease was thought to act as a depressant upon the central nervous system, some of the after-effects of influenza were psychological. Harvey Cushing noted in 1906 that a victim was apt to be quarrelsome, irritable, despondent, and have a hopelessness of spirit.

Imagine a nation of irritable and quarrelsome people, living through a period of social, political, and economic stress! Were the Red Scare excesses in some measure the result of a nation in a less-than-generous mood? Did the race riots and spate of strikes in the post-war period reflect to some degree the quarrelsomeness associated with influenza? Was the universal apathy and hopelessness of spirit commented upon by the noted editor of the Emporia Gazette, William Allen White, partly physically-induced? The United States, like the rest of the world, was clearly out-of-sorts at the end of the second decade of the twentieth century. Its citizens' sick minds and sick bodies needed healing, perhaps more than at any other time in the nation's history.

Still, nearly a century after the devastating pandemic of 1918, many questions remain unanswered. The main question of course remains the same: Can we expect a pandemic similar to the one which occurred in 1918 to strike the world again? Global influenza pandemics did occur in 1957 and again in 1968. According to Jamie Shreeve, those who died seemed to be the young, the old and those with chronic conditions.[1] The number of fatalities in 1957 was about 2 million and in 1968 approximately 700,000. The exact death toll figures of the 1918 pandemic are never likely to be known with complete accuracy, but scholarly estimates vary between 20 to 50 and even 100 million.[2]

Among the theories about the origin of the pandemic is that of the eminent British scientist, Professor John S. Oxford, who initially postulated that the 1918 influenza virus spread eastward to China from Europe.[3] He described an outbreak of a strikingly similar respiratory disease, then known as "purulent bronchitis," with rapid onset and spreadability and high mortality, in young soldiers in the British base camp at Etaples, France during the winter of 1916-1917. Victims exhibited the same symptoms of "heliotrope cyanosis" that was so characteristic of those who died during the autumn wave of the 1918 pandemic. According to Oxford, pathologists who performed the autopsies on these soldiers subsequently agreed that this—and the lethal 1918 pandemic influenza—were one and the same. In spite of the fact that no samples are available from those autopsies for verification of the viral gene sequences, Oxford has continued to develop this hypothesis and, in early 2005, argued that:

> The Etaples camp had the necessary mixture of factors for emergence of pandemic influenza including overcrowding (with 100,000 soldiers daily changing), live pigs and nearby live geese, duck and chicken markets, horses and an additional factor 24 gases (some of them mutagenic) used in large 100 ton quantities to contaminate soldiers and the landscape. The final trigger for the ensuing pandemic was the return of millions of soldiers to their homelands around the entire world in the autumn of 1918.[4]

Certainly, Oxford's hypothesis is a plausible one. The overcrowded conditions in the camps, the proximity of birds, mammals and humans and the presence of mutagenic gases that are now known to facilitate changes in the sequence of genes, were all factors that would provide a highly permissive environment for the development of a novel strain of a virus with pandemic potential.

Another theory places the origin of the pandemic in the United States itself. In 2004, best-selling author and historian John M. Barry, highlighted a previously unknown—and again remarkably similar—epidemic of influenza, which occurred during January and February of 1918 in Haskell County, Kansas, an isolated, and notably sparsely populated, rural community three hundred miles west of Camp Funston (Kansas). Like the outbreak in Etaples, the epidemic in Haskell County subsided as suddenly as it began, but a local physician, Dr. Loring Miner, considered the outbreak sufficiently remarkable to report it to the United States Public Health Service. Barry notes that all Army personnel from the county reported to Camp Funston for training, many between February 26 and March 2, 1918. He even mentions the specific case of one Ernest Elliot, who was reported by the *Santa Fe Monitor* to have left Haskell for a visit to his brother at Funston, just as his son, Mertin, fell ill with pneumonia. According to Barry and some others, the first cases of influenza were reported at Camp Funston on March 4, 1918.[5] Again, as for Etaples, autopsy samples are unavailable from Haskell, so Barry's theory cannot be further substantiated.

What we know of influenza today is that the strain responsible for so many deaths in the fall of 1918 was indeed lethal. We know this thanks to the extraordinary and persistent efforts of men like the ever-curious pathologist Johan Hultin, research pathologist Jeffrey Taubenberger of the Armed Forces Institute of Pathology, and microbiologist Terrence Tumpey at the Centers for Disease Control in Atlanta. As the science journalist Jamie Shreeve and others have noted, Swedish-born Johan Hultin's involvement started when he was a twenty-five year old graduate student at the University of Iowa, probably during the academic year 1949-50.

Hultin was seeking an interesting topic for his doctoral thesis. He learned of the devastating loss of seventy-two inhabitants that was suffered by Teller Mission, a tiny Inuit village in Alaska, during the pandemic in November 1918. Hultin was so struck by the stories that he, along with two colleagues, visited the Mission in 1951, hoping that the lungs of some of the victims buried in the Alaskan permafrost would contain enough frozen virus to set up live cultures. After obtaining permission from the Inuit tribal elders to excavate the graves, he recovered tissue specimens from the frozen remains of several victims. Much to Hultin's disappointment, his attempts to establish live cultures were unsuccessful. The failure probably spared him from exposing himself and others to the deadly virus. Today such dangerous viruses are handled only in laboratories designed to keep them safely contained from contact with humans. However, handled correctly, it was hoped that if the genetic sequence of the viral genes could be obtained, it would answer some of the longstanding questions posed by the 1918 pandemic.

Efforts to learn more about the virus are today being pioneered by a group headed by Taubenberger at the Armed Forces Institute of Pathology in Rockville, Maryland. Sophisticated scientific techniques—and some luck—have combined to allow this group to make extraordinary advances in the understanding of the 1918 pandemic influenza virus.

Their quest began with the examination of autopsy samples from 1918 flu victims stored at the Institute. Influenza virus does not normally persist in the lungs beyond three days after infection; thus, in order to maximize their chances of finding virus in the samples, they focused on those victims who had succumbed during the first few days of illness. As an RNA virus, the genetic material of influenza is very fragile. These samples, preserved eighty years earlier by traditional methods, posed an enormous challenge to the scientists, who had to refine their extraction techniques in order to have a chance of recovering a sample of the viral RNA that could provide useful information.

Their persistence paid off, however, when in 1996, a lung sample from a young soldier who had been a victim of influenza in

September 1918 at Fort Jackson, South Carolina, yielded the first fragments of five—out of the eight—genes from the 1918 virus to be sequenced. A year later, tissue from a second victim, who had also died in September 1918, at Camp Upton, New York, was also found to contain the virus, and allowed confirmation of the initial results.

It was at that point that the researchers got their lucky break. Johan Hultin, by now retired from his long career as a pathologist in San Francisco, had maintained his interest in the influenza pandemic. When he read of the results from Taubenberger's group he felt compelled to offer to return to the Mission (now renamed the "Brevig Mission") in the hope that some of the lungs of the victims buried in the permafrost would provide further samples from which genetic information could be recovered. Permission was granted for a second exhumation, and when it was respectfully and painstakingly carried out, one of the samples, obtained from a female victim affectionately named Lucy, provided enough viral material to complete the remaining sequence of the viral genes. That finding, together with further sequences recovered concurrently from British autopsy samples, has confirmed that the virus wreaking havoc on each side of the Atlantic was identical.[6]

Jeffrey Taubenberger and his team have spent considerable time since that work scrutinizing the sequences of the 1918 genes and comparing them with other influenza strains. Having believed for some time that the virus, although containing some avian elements, had been modified during passage through an intermediary such as swine, the team has concluded that the virus arose suddenly and as a result of direct bird-to-human infection by means of an adaptation of an avian influenza strain to infect humans. Their findings are disputed by other groups—including Mark J. Gibbs and Adrian J. Gibbs of the Australian National University, who believe that the results indicate that the virus may have evolved in *mammals*, instead of birds—before the beginning of the pandemic through the gene shuffling mechanism generally referred to as reassortment.[7] The continued debate is of supreme importance from the point of view of global surveillance, which largely focuses on avian influenza. If it is determined that—instead of jumping from birds to humans, the virus instead is transmitted from mammals to humans—then surveillance would have to be expanded to include a broader range of species to be effective.

Having obtained the full genetic sequence of the 1918 virus, Taubenberger and his colleagues wished to examine the properties associated with its extraordinary virulence. An in-depth examination of the genetic sequence was conducted, bearing in mind the specific sequence motifs that have been found to contribute to infectivity and virulence in other pandemic strains and those that circulate in non-pandemic years. During years of research into influenza, scientists have been able to link certain genetic sequences with the tricks that influenza viruses can use to get around host defenses and turn the body's immune system against itself.

For example, to become active in the cells, the HA protein must be cleaved into two pieces. In general, influenza viruses use a single specific enzyme found in the host's own tissues to do this. However, some strains have changes that allow this cleavage by a broader range of the host's enzymes, while others have dispensed with the need for host enzymes by changing to a host-independent cleavage mechanism.[8] But the 1918 virus contained no known sequence motifs that would immediately explain its extraordinary killing power, suggesting that the genes concealed either a single, previously unidentified motif that was responsible for its high level of virulence, or that a number of coordinated features of the virus were at play.

If answers were to be found, experiments with live virus were more likely to provide them, and since not one single specimen had ever been successfully isolated, the team needed to take a different approach. Taubenberger and his group joined forces with researchers from the Centers for Disease Control and Prevention, Mount Sinai School of Medicine and the US Department of

Agriculture (USDA) Poultry Research Laboratory. Working under stringent safety conditions and using an ultra modern technique called plasmid-based reverse genetics, the group initially created viral strains in which one or more of the genes in a contemporary H1N1 strain was replaced with the 1918 genes – these are termed hybrid viruses. In later experiments, a virus containing the full 1918 sequence was generated. These viruses were then used to infect mice and the virulence of the contemporary strains, the hybrids, and the full 1918 virus was compared.

In all of the experiments, the 1918 virus lived up to its reputation: it caused mortality and destruction of the mouse lung tissue that mirrored the pathologists' findings in the lungs of the 1918 victims. The experiments also showed that the 1918 virus reproduced at least one hundred-fold, and sometimes many thousand-fold faster, far more successfully than any of the hybrid or contemporary strains, resulting in overwhelmingly large numbers of viral particles in the lung tissue. To achieve such a rapid growth rate, cooperation between the 1918 HA and 1918 polymerase genes seemed to be an absolute requirement. While it is thought that viruses containing the 1918 NS1 gene were more effective than other strains at blocking the hosts type I interferon system—the early warning system that the body uses to activate the immune response to infection—the 1918 HA gene was necessary for development of the most severe damage to the lung tissue, resulting in an intensive immune response. Furthermore, even though the known motifs for host-independent HA cleavage were not present in the 1918 virus, it was clear that the HA protein was activated by a previously uncharacterized mechanism. The authors concluded that:

> The constellation of all eight genes together make an exceptionally virulent virus in the model systems examined. In fact, no other human influenza viruses that have been tested show a similar pathogenicity for mice…This information provides a partial explanation for what made this virus so lethal.[9]

The mice died! And that was the final proof that influenza could kill and was not just a three day minor annoyance, a view that was still held by some physicians in the 1970s and 1980s. In essence, it would seem that in 1918, a supremely well-adapted influenza virus came into existence, undoubtedly helped by the extremely permissive conditions in which it found itself. In other words, a combination of chance and environment contributed to the creation of a powerful killer virus. Because no exhumations were done on any victims of the previous winter and spring, we cannot be certain the recently recreated pandemic virus was not in circulation before the fall of 1918. Perhaps some intrepid scientist will one day find a way to express RNA samples from the earlier victims.

Undoubtedly, Taubenberger's team and their collaborators will continue their experiments with the 1918 strain, and hopefully these will provide even more vital information that will be helpful in protecting the world from a similar event in the future.

The truth of the matter is that medical professionals were helpless bystanders in the face of the 1918 pandemic. Historians today might well warn against the same "scientific triumphalism" that accompanied the successful identification of many bacterial infections in the late nineteenth and early twentieth centuries, and which was dealt such a bitter blow by the Spanish flu. The 1928 discovery of penicillin by Alexander Fleming, a Scottish biologist and pharmacologist, along with the subsequent advances during the twentieth century in the development of antibiotic and antiviral drugs, and the "eradication" of smallpox and polio, led to a renewed illusion of a world relatively free of infectious diseases, which persisted until the advent of AIDS in the 1980s.[10] Our struggles against the AIDS virus have renewed our respect for such diseases, but an even more acute reminder of our vulnerability was the outbreak of Severe Acute Respiratory Syndrome (SARS) in 2003.

It is important to remember that, like ourselves, microbes must battle for survival, and to do this in today's world, they need to equip themselves to circumvent the efforts we have made to overcome them. The emergence of a new strain of pandemic influenza from a source in nature is a distinct possibility. And, in light of the frequent reports of human infection with avian influenza strains, some say it is inevitable that another pandemic will occur. There are also fears that the sophisticated techniques used by scientists for the public good could be used for the purposes of bioterrorism.[11]

There is also the possibility of accidental release, as demonstrated by the shipping by courier of the 1957 pandemic strain by a biotechnology company to more than 6,000 laboratories worldwide as part of an influenza test kit in 2005. In that case, the company was alerted of its error by an employee in the laboratory of one of the customers, who recognized that the potentially deadly viral strain had been sent out in the kits. Following the discovery, laboratories worldwide destroyed the samples, but the incident raised concerns as to how such a mistake could have occurred, and the potential threat it had posed to public health. In the modern world, the spread of a disease such as influenza would be almost instantaneous around the globe. As such, we must use every weapon in our armory to avoid the exposure of the human race to an unfamiliar and potentially deadly virus.

The remainder of this chapter describes the current interest in the avian H5N1 influenza strain, which, it is feared, has the potential to acquire the mutations it needs to gain a foothold in the human population. There is also discussion of the state of global surveillance and the prophylactic measures that are being put in place against such an eventuality.

Three international agencies coordinate the global surveillance effort for influenza. The World Health Organization monitors human cases, while the World Organization for Animal Health (OIE), and the Food and Agriculture Organization (FAO) collect reports on outbreaks in birds and other animals. These agencies are, in turn, supported by a network of laboratories that isolate and test specimens recovered. There is growing concern over the increasing frequency of direct bird-to-human influenza transmission during the last decade, and outbreaks caused by several different subtypes including H7N7, H9N2, H7N3, H10N7 and H5N1 have been recorded.[12] While infection of humans by avian influenza is not thought to be a novel phenomenon, heightened influenza awareness on a global scale has most likely put the spotlight on such events. Nonetheless, the WHO has noted that currently the H5N1 avian influenza virus is infecting a broader range of both avian and non-avian species, and already the virus is under heavy scrutiny to determine the level of pandemic threat it poses to humans.[13]

Between the start of the latest outbreak of H5N1 in Vietnam in 2003 and February 2007, 275 human cases of H5N1 influenza were reported, with 167 fatalities.[14] So far the fatality rate in humans has been high (between fifty-five to fifty-nine percent) and the most frequently affected have been those between five and twenty-three years.[15] Even if the fatality rates were to fall dramatically, which is normally the trade-off that influenza—crossing the species barrier—has to make to allow transmissibility between humans, H5N1 would still appear to represent a potential threat at least as great as the 1918 pandemic.[16]

Using the lessons that have been learned from examination of the 1918 and other contemporary influenza strains, scientists at the Scripps Institute in California, working together with Taubenberger and his colleagues, are examining the H5N1 gene sequences and relating these to the potential ability of the currently circulating strains to infect humans.[17] Initial findings suggest that the H5N1 strains isolated so far from humans in 1997 in Hong Kong and 2004 in Vietnam have already acquired one of the changes predicted to be important to the ability of the virus to infect humans. Although some of the most recent cases, particularly in Indonesia, are suspected of being human-to-human transmission, they are thought to be the result of close and prolonged exposure of family members nursing sick relatives. This reflects the known difficulty for viruses to make the jump between species and go on to spread efficiently amongst the new species. At the time of writing, the viral sequence has still not developed the further changes that are necessary to allow efficient human-to-human transmission.[18] It is believed that monitoring the rate at which these changes to the viral sequence are acquired may enable scientists to track viruses years before they develop the capacity to replicate with high efficiency in humans.[19]

Of great concern is the fact that the H5N1 Vietnam 2004 HA protein is structurally more similar to the 1918 and other human hemagglutinins than are many avian HA proteins.[20] Most recently, the Scripps researchers have used modern microarray technology to examine in detail the binding of virus to various human and avian binding site glycoproteins. The microarrays will be invaluable in monitoring the evolution of influenza strains as they acquire the ability to overcome the species barrier.[21] Much commercial energy is also being put into the development of diagnostic tests that can rapidly identify the HA and NA subtype of influenza, which would allow a more immediate response to a fresh outbreak.[22]

In the absence of any effective antiviral vaccine, antiviral drugs or antibiotics to combat the secondary infections, the 1918 pandemic raged unchecked. In today's world, expert opinions differ on the relative benefits and the appropriate use of each in the event of a possible global pandemic. The latest WHO guidelines recognize:

> ....*a period on the cusp of a pandemic when such a strain may be intercepted and restrained, if not stamped out....*[23]

Powerful mathematical modeling computer programs which use massive quantities of data collected from around the world have been developed to accurately simulate the spread of influenza in pandemic form. In these model systems, the effect of any factor—

air travel, public health control measures or drug interventions on the likely spread of the virus and the economic impacts—can be examined. Clearly the response to an outbreak of a new potential pandemic influenza strain would have to be exceptionally swift. During the SARS epidemic that emerged in China in 2003, where the time from exposure of a victim to becoming infectious was around ten days, the virus could be contained by tracing and isolating those who had been in contact with the victim before they, too, became infectious. In contrast, influenza victims begin showing symptoms and shedding infectious particles in as few as two days post-infection, so it is unlikely that contact tracing and isolation alone would be effective.[24]

A group at Imperial College, London, headed by mathematical biologist, Neil M. Ferguson, is carrying out sophisticated predictive modeling of influenza pandemics. All such models are based on assumptions about the behavior of the virus, especially the reproductive number R(0), and how quickly the cases are reported. Ferguson's models, based on the demographics and geography of Thailand, predict that, given sufficient quantities of antiviral drugs and even a low efficiency vaccine, there would be a potential window of about 30 days from the initial person-to-person transmission in which the containment of a pandemic could be achieved.[25] Biostatistician Ira Longini, Jr. and colleagues at Emory University in Atlanta, have carried out other mathematical modeling experiments which have included prophylactic vaccination of the community in advance of an outbreak, and have found that even better outcomes were predicted.[26] They advise that any available vaccine should be used for prevention in the region where human adapted virus is likely to emerge, even if less vaccine would then be available for the inhabitants of the countries which provided it.[27]

Nonetheless, the WHO still has concern about the reliability of surveillance and also social customs in some parts of Asia; the latter has sometimes prohibited autopsies and resulted in lengthy delays before confirmation of human H5N1 cases. Undoubtedly, developing countries are at risk of being hardest hit by a pandemic and inadequate surveillance measures may result in failure of containment should a pandemic arise.

In general, models have concluded that global travel restrictions would have surprisingly little effect unless almost all travel ceases very soon after epidemics are detected, and that local measures are likely to be more effective.[28] Interestingly, though, a recent study examined the only practical instance of a large-scale air travel restriction—the flight ban in the United States after the terrorist attack on September 11, 2001. That study showed that the decrease in air travel was associated with a delayed and prolonged influenza season. Further modeling studies will be informed by this evidence.[29]

Neil M. Ferguson and his colleagues at the Imperial College of London, continue to produce models—based on data from the United Kingdom and United States—that examine approaches that might be worthy of adoption if containment of a novel influenza strain at the source fails. The models are complex and include such social distancing measures as school closures, border restrictions, case isolation and household quarantine.[30] Again, given enough antiviral drugs and a low efficacy vaccine, attack rates may be controllable. Of course, the effectiveness of any measure also depends on the characteristics of the particular pandemic strain.

Amantadines, antiviral drugs that have been given to poultry in parts of Asia, are useful in the treatment of some H5N1 strains that have infected humans, but their application may be limited by the development of resistance. All influenza strains tested so far, including a number of Taubenberger's reconstructed viruses, containing proteins from the 1918 strain and H5N1, are susceptible to modern antiviral neuraminidase inhibitor drugs (oseltamivir [Tamiflu™] and zanamivir [Relenza™]) when tested in mice.[31] These drugs could, in theory, be used prophylactically to prevent the spread of infection in families and communities, where an eighty to ninety percent protection has been documented.[32]

However, the long-term effects of prolonged use of any such drugs have not been tested and could cause unforeseen problems. For treatment of influenza, the drugs have to be taken within 48 hours of the appearance of symptoms.

It is proposed that these antiviral drugs could be stockpiled in preparation for an influenza pandemic, and indeed some administrations have already made this decision. Antivirals will be the front line of defense until a suitable vaccine can be developed, although supplies will undoubtedly be under severe pressure. Some experts caution against the overuse of such drugs, because of the threat that drug-resistant viral strains will develop; this has recently been observed to occur even during treatment.[33] The mutant strains of influenza that have developed so far are compromised, less virulent than their drug-sensitive parents and spread less easily.[34] Nonetheless, because of the adaptability of the influenza virus, judicious use of antiviral drugs is essential to ensure their effectiveness as a first line of defense in the next and future pandemics, and a careful watch is being kept on the emergence of drug-resistant strains.[35]

Another antiviral, peramivir, which has a similar mode of action, is claimed to be more potent than both oseltamivir and zanamivir, and could be produced more rapidly and less expensively. That drug will hopefully soon be available for administration intravenously to hospitalized influenza victims. In initial tests the drug has shown efficacy even against some strains of influenza that have developed resistance to oseltamivir and zanamivir.[36]

The risks of developing drug resistant mutants, coupled with the expense of providing these treatments on a global scale, have fueled the search for new and potentially less expensive anti-influenza drugs. Particularly attractive are those which are less likely to be affected by the hypermutability of the virus; for example: an inhalant preparation has been developed, which acts by removing the influenza viral receptors—sialic acids—from the host cells. The preparation works for both the receptors used by avian and human influenza strains, and preliminary tests have shown long-lasting effects, with low toxicity and high efficacy in both prevention and treatment.[37] Another group has developed a product that mimics the sialic acid target receptor structure, which then binds to the virus, blocking its sialidase activity.[38] There is a risk that full clinical trials of novel products will not be completed on time should a fresh pandemic arise very soon, and difficult decisions may need to be taken about using them to treat victims.

Antibiotics were unavailable in 1918, and there is no data that can discriminate between the direct victims of influenza and those who died from secondary infections. Data is available from the 1968 pandemic, showing that Staphylococcus aureus caused twenty-six percent of the infections, and Streptococcus pneumoniae, forty-eight percent.[39] Universal prophylactic antibiotic use is not acceptable, because it is likely to encourage antibiotic resistance, and current guidelines on managing influenza restrict antibiotic treatment to people with signs and symptoms of pneumonia, especially the very young and very old and those with underlying diseases. Some review of these guidelines may be necessary, depending on the age range affected by any new pandemic—5 to 23 years of age for H5N1, for example. A particular challenge will be the emergent threat of community acquired methicillin-resistant Staphylococcus aureus (CA-MRSA). Since individuals carrying such infections may be at particular risk of severe complications during an influenza pandemic, recently developed rapid diagnostic tests that can detect carriers of S. aureus could be useful in the identification of patients at increased risk for secondary pneumonia.[40]

Seasonal vaccination for influenza is now recommended, and is indeed routine for at-risk groups, although emergency plans would need to be put into place to coordinate mass vaccination on the level needed to control an influenza pandemic. Lessons have undoubtedly been learned from one previous experience with such a program. In January 1976, four Army recruits at Fort Dix, New Jersey were found to be sick with influenza. The virus that was isolated was called swine flu and was thought to be similar to the 1918 influenza strain.

The U.S. Public Health Service, in partnership with the Centers for Disease Control and Prevention (CDC), and backed by a panel of experts, recommended a universal immunization campaign. A $135 million emergency fund was then granted for the preparation of the vaccine, which was to be developed and production overseen by the CDC before the fall of 1976. Vaccination began on October 1, 1976, and within ten weeks, almost 50 million Americans had received the vaccine. In this particular instance, no epidemic influenza was seen, so it appears that the efforts were wasted. Also, while the exercise demonstrated the feasibility of such a program of vaccination, the story had a somewhat unfortunate ending in that, about eight weeks into the campaign, cases of a rare, paralytic condition known as Guillain-Barré Syndrome began to appear, and a causal link to the vaccine seemed clear. By mid-December 1976, the vaccination program was suspended.[41]

Current surveillance—if carried out effectively by all nations—and available technologies are capable of providing sufficient information to prevent such a response to another red herring influenza strain. Clinical trials of any new vaccine will need to be carefully conducted, especially in view of the time pressures that are likely to be imposed by the demands of a world in the grip of pandemic influenza. Adverse responses to any vaccine will always be a risk that must be balanced against the benefits to public health that prevention of influenza would bring, but careful monitoring and immediate reporting of such responses must be an essential part of any mass immunization program.

Many believe that even a vaccine with limited effectiveness would be of benefit in the fight against a global influenza pandemic.[42] As far as H5N1 is concerned, such a vaccine has been produced using a seed vaccine developed from the 2004 Vietnam strain. Production of an effective H5N1 vaccine has proved particularly challenging, and any vaccines raised so far have required a relatively high dose to produce a response. This is a problem as there is a limited global capacity for vaccine manufacture.[43] While stockpiling of vaccine in advance of a pandemic is an option, doing so poses yet other problems. Total worldwide production of flu vaccine amounts to roughly 300 million doses a year, all of which are currently provided to high-risk groups.[44] Contamination in manufacturing plants is also a risk, such as the one which halted production in a British facility in 2004, and which—in turn—placed added pressure on European and United States facilities. There are plans to increase global production, and some manufacturers are getting ready to build new facilities, but they may not be operating either at full capacity, or the new plants may not even have begun production, should a pandemic occur in the next few years.

At present, the constitution of the vaccine is changed each year when the season's circulating strains have been identified. As noted by Pascale Wortley of the CDC's National Immunization Program, a manufacturing plant will produce vaccine against only one strain at a time (the final product is a combination of vaccines against several current strains). If a new pandemic strain emerged, manufacturers whose plants were already busy with the seasonal vaccines, may have to make a choice whether to switch from the annual vaccine to the pandemic one.[45]

Vaccine against only one strain at a time can be produced in a vaccine plant, so a choice would have to be made whether to switch from the annual vaccine to the pandemic one. Furthermore, the shelf life of the vaccine is limited and—at the present rate of production—supply would struggle to fulfill the demand of countries wishing to stockpile at the level required for pandemic preparedness. Finally, manufacturers would see the exclusive prophylactic production of a vaccine against a predicted pandemic as an enormous financial risk unless the contracts included liability clauses or guaranteed purchases.

Without a doubt, research that is aiming to develop new technologies for vaccine production will overcome some of these hurdles – whether this will happen soon enough for the next pandemic is not certain.[46] Given the fact that multiple variants of influenza virus will circulate simultaneously, a truly efficient vaccine for a pandemic strain could be produced only once it had emerged, and at the present rate of production, specific vaccines would still take approximately six months to produce. For effective immunization, recipients of a vaccine against a previously unencountered pandemic strain would require a first shot, followed by a booster dose, so time would be required to develop a full immune response. Other prophylactic measures, such as the controlled and targeted use of anti-viral drugs and antibiotics, and good public health management, would be needed to stall the progress of the virus to give time for vaccine production. Much research is now focusing on faster ways to produce vaccines.

In public health terms, the importance in pandemic planning of the emergency provision of hospitals with sufficient medical and nursing services cannot be overstated. Such services, which are so vital—but were so overstretched during the 1918 pandemic—need to be able to cope in the best possible way with the estimated numbers of potential hospitalizations that would result from a global pandemic. A Princeton University Policy Research Institute assessment noted that in a December 2006 Associated Press review of state preparedness plans, "half the states would run out of hospital beds within two weeks in just a moderate flu pandemic and 40 [states would] face a nursing shortage."[47]

One effective control measure that can be taken against avian influenza is the isolation and culling of infected fowl as has been practiced in China, Vietnam and Thailand in response to avian flu outbreaks. The proximity of poultry, pigs and humans in densely settled rural areas is being addressed by agricultural reforms in China.[48] It is cause for concern therefore that this practice is being reversed in the United States as the animal industry continues to develop highly dense animal population feed lot concepts for raising swine and poultry near populated regions.[49] An outbreak of

H5N1 avian influenza in Suffolk, England in early 2007 is under investigation by the British Department for Environment, Food and Rural Affairs, for potential links with imported poultry and poultry products from a source in Europe. The outbreak led to the slaughter of 160,000 turkeys at the infected plant, and highlights the fact that the movement of such products around the world requires ever more careful monitoring. Moreover, the role of migratory birds in the spread of avian influenza is, as yet, an unknown quantity, but recently, dead birds carrying the H5N1 virus have been found in the UK. Monitoring of migratory bird populations is also a vital part of the prevention effort.

Sharing information within the science community can sometimes be slow, as researchers try to protect their intellectual property to make sure they get the credit for their findings. However, because in the case of an influenza pandemic such delays could be disastrous; influenza researchers recently formed a consortium called the Global Initiative on Sharing Avian Influenza Data (GISAID), which encourages scientists to deposit findings about the virus in databases such as the United States-based *Genbank* within six months of discovery. But, as some researchers point out, six months is still a very long time in the face of an influenza pandemic.[50]

Except for its severity, the 1918-1920 influenza pandemic was similar to previous and subsequent pandemics that have marched around the globe in search of victims. Results of experiments also demonstrate that recombinant influenza viruses with genetic material from the 1918 virus appear "as sensitive as other typical virus strains" to FDA-approved drugs such as rimantadine and oseltamivir.[51]

However, in regard to its severity, certain factors—such as the sheer number of individuals worldwide who became clinically ill from the virus, the higher percentage of severe, complicated respiratory tract infections, the impact of the virus on younger members of the population, especially those aged twenty-to-forty, and the fact that the virus came in waves—appear largely responsible for the exhorbitant mortality rate of the 1918 influenza pandemic. A mortality rate, five to *twenty* times higher than usual! And, as Jeffrey Taubenberger and David Morens point out, the impact of the pandemic was not limited to 1918-1919.

In their capstone paper, "1918 Influenza: The Mother of All Pandemics," published in *Emerging Infectious Disease*, they wrote:

> *Until we can ascertain which...factors gave rise to the mortality patterns observed and learn more about the formation of the [1918] pandemic, [our] predictions are only educated guesses. We can only conclude that since it happened once, analogous conditions could lead to an equally devestating pandemic.*
>
> *Like the 1918 virus, H5N1 is an avian virus, though a distantly related one. [And while] the evolutionary path that led to pandemic emergence in 1918 is entirely unknown, it appears to be different in many respects from the current situation with H5N1. There are no historical data...for establishing that a pandemic 'precursor' virus caused a highly pathogenic outbreak in domestic poultry, and no highly pathogenic avian influenza (HPAI) virus, including H5N1...has ever been known to cause a major human epidemic, let alone a pandemic. [Further], while data bearing on influenza virus human cell adaptation (e.g., receptor binding) are beginning to be understood at the molecular level, the basis for viral adaptation to efficient human-to-human spread, the chief prerequisite for pandemic emergence, is [still] unknown for any influenza virus. The 1918 influenza virus acquired this trait, but we do not know how, and we currently have no way of knowing whether H5N1 viruses are now on a parallel process of acquiring human-to-human transmissibility...*
>
> *Even with modern antiviral and antibacterial drugs, vaccines, and prevention knowledge, the return of a pandemic virus equivalent in pathogenicity to the virus of 1918 would likely kill >100 million people worldwide. [And], a pandemic virus with*

the alleged pathogenic potential of some recent H5N1 outbreaks could cause substantially more deaths.[52]

The 1918 pandemic influenza descended upon an un-suspecting world. Today, global surveillance and technology may have given us the chance to prevent such a pandemic from ever again taking us by complete surprise. Still, we must treat this microscopic 'mass murderer' with the utmost respect and never doubt its exceptional ability to adapt, taking advantage of permissive conditions where it can, and overcome adverse conditions to develop resistance to treatments that destroy it when it must.

However, with careful management, humanitarian support and a huge amount of cooperative local, national and international effort, there is still the chance that we can reduce, and even possibly minimize the impact of a new pandemic.

Or, so we hope.

A Cruel Wind:
Pandemic Flu in America, 1918-1920

Notes/
Select Bibliography

Notes

CHAPTER 1: THE RIDDLE OF INFLUENZA

1. John F. Fulton, *Harvey Cushing: A Biography* (Springfield, Ill.: Charles C. Thomas, Publishers, 1946), 251.

2. See Fulton, pp. 435-520, 710-14; *Harvey Cushing, From A Surgeon's Journal 1915-1918* (Boston: Little, Brown, 1934), 413-511; and W.G. MacCallum, "Biographical Memoir of Harvey Cushing," in *Biographical Memoirs of the National Academy of Sciences of the United States of America*, vol. 23 (Washington, D.C.: National Academy of Sciences, 1943), 49-70.

3. U.S. Department of the Army, *The Medical Department of the United States Army in the World War*, by M.W. Ireland, vol. 9: *Communicable and Other Diseases*, by Joseph F. Siler (Washington, D.C.: U.S. Government Printing Office, 1928), 155.

4. Albert W. Crosby, *America's Forgotten Pandemic: The Influenza of 1918*, 2d ed. (Cambridge: Cambridge UP, 2003), 5.

5. John F. Brundage, "Interactions Between Influenza and Bacterial Respiratory Pathogens: Implications for Pandemic Preparedness," *Lancet Infectious Diseases* 6, no. 5 (May 2006): 303-12.

6. Masato Tashiro, Pawel S. Ciborowski, Hans Dieter Klenk, Gerhard Pulverer, and Rudolf Rott, "Role of Staphylococcus Protease in the Development of Influenza Pneumonia," *Nature* 325, 5 February 1987, 536-37.

7. Jonathan A. McCullers, "Insights into the Interaction Between Influenza Virus and Pneumococcus," *Clinical Microbiology Reviews* 19, no. 3 (July 2006): 571-82.

8. Graham Selby Wilson and A. Ashley Miles, *Topley and Wilson's Principles of Bacteriology and Immunology*, 2 vols. 5th ed., (London: Edward Arnold, 1966), 1164.

9. Ibid.

10. Ronald Eccles, "Understanding the Symptoms of the Common Cold and Influenza," *Lancet Infectious Diseases*

5, no. 11 (November 2005): 718-725; Mongkol Uiprasertkul, Pilaipan Puthavathana, Kantima Sangsiriwut, Phisanu Pooruk, Kanittar Srisook, Malik Peiris, John M. Nicholls, Kulkanya Chokephaibulkit, Nirun Vanprapar, and Prasert Auewarakul, "Influenza A H5N1 Replication Sites in Humans" *Emerging Infectious Diseases* 11, no. 7 (July 2005): 1036-41.

11. *Stedman's Medical Dictionary for the Health Professions and Nursing.* Illus. 5th ed. (Philadelphia: Lippincott Williams & Wilkins, 2005), 1564.

12. Vernon Knight and Julius A. Kasel, "Influenza Viruses," in *Viral and Mycoplasmal Infections of the Respiratory Tract*, ed. Vernon Knight (Philadelphia: Lea & Febinger, 1973), 99.

13. Ibid.

14. Jeffery K. Taubenberger, Ann H. Reid and Thomas G. Fanning, "Capturing a Killer Flu Virus," *Scientific American* 292, no 1 (January 2005): 62-71

15. Vernon Knight, pp. 95-100.

16. Jeffery K. Taubenberger, "Chasing the Elusive 1918 Virus: Preparing for the Future by Examining the Past," in *The Threat of Pandemic Influenza, Are we Ready?: Workshop Summary*, eds. Stacey L. Knobler, Alison Mack, Adel Mahmoud, and Stanley M. Lemon (Washington, D.C.: National Academics Press, 2005); Ann H. Reid and Jeffery K. Taubenberger, "The Origin of the 1918 Pandemic Influenza Virus: A Continuing Enigma," *Journal of General Virology* 84, pt. 9 (September 2003): 2285-92; Terrence M. Tumpey, Christopher F. Basler, Patricia V. Aguilar, Hui Zeng, Alicia Solorzano, David E. Swayne, Nancy J. Cox, Jacqueline M. Katz, Jeffrey

K. Taubenberger, Peter Palese, Adolofo Garcia-Sastre, "Characterization of the Reconstructed 1918 Spanish Influenza Pandemic Virus," *Science* 310 no. 5745, 7 October 2005, 77-80; Gary K. Geiss, Mirella Salvatore, Terrence M. Tumpey, Victoria S. Carter, Xiuyan Wang, Christopher F. Basler, Jeffrey K. Taubenberger, Roger E. Bumgarner, Peter Palese, Michael G. Katze, Adolofo Garcia-Sastre, "Cellular Transcriptional Profiling in Influenza A Virus-infected Lung Epithelial Cells: The Role of the Nonstructural NS1 Protein in the Evasion of the Host Innate Defense and its Potential Contribution to Pandemic Influenza," *Proceedings of the National Academy of Sciences of the United States of America* 99, no. 16, 6 August 2002, 10736-41.

17. Taubenberger et al., 2005.

18. Leslie Hoyle, *The Influenza Viruses*, vol. 4 of *Virology Monographs: Continuing Handbook of Virus Research*, ed. by S. Gard, C. Hallauer, and H. F. Meyer (New York: Springer-Verlag, 1968), 114.

19. Ibid., 206.

20. Adolfo Garcia-Sastre, "Antiviral Response in Pandemic Influenza Viruses," *Emerging Infectious Diseases* 12, no. 1 (January 2006): 44-47.

21. Julie Talon, Curt M. Horvath, Rosalind Polley, Christopher F. Basler, Thomas F. Muster, Peter Palese, Adolfo Garcia-Sastre, "Activation of Interferon Regulatory Factor 3 is Inhibited by the Influenza A Virus NS1 Protein," *Journal of Virology* 74, no. 17 (September 2000): 7989-7996

22. Weisan Chen, Paul A. Calvo, Daniela Malide, James Gibbs, Ulrich Schubert, Igor Bacik, Sameh Basta,

et al., "A Novel Influenza A Virus Mitochondrial Protein that Induces Cell Death," *Nature Medicine* 7 (2001): 1306-12; R. Joel Lowy, "Influenza Virus Induction of Apoptosis by Intrinsic and Extrinsic Mechanisms," *International Reviews of Immunology* 22, nos. 5-6, (2003): 425-449.

23. William A. Carter and Erik De Clercq, "Viral Infection and Host Defense," *Science* 186 no. 4170, 27 December 1974, 1172-78.

24. Darwyn Kobasa, Ayato Takada, Kyoko Shinya, Masato Hatta, Peter Halfmann, Steven Theriault, Hirishi Suzuki, et al., "Enhanced Virulence of Influenza A Viruses with the Haemagglutinin of the 1918 Pandemic Virus," *Nature* 431, 7 October 2004, 703-707; Michael T. Osterholm, "Preparing for the Next Pandemic," *New England Journal of Medicine* 352, no. 18, 5 May 2005, 1839-42.

25. Hoyle, p. 211; William M. Marine and Wilton M. Workman, "Hong Kong Influenza Immunologic Recapitulation," *American Journal of Epidemiology* 90, no. 5 (1969): 406-415.

26. See both Hoyle, Ibid., and Knight, 100-01.

27. Lone Simonsen, Thomas A. Reichert, and Mark A. Miller. In *Options for the Control of Influenza V*, ed. Yoshihiro Kawaoka. International Congress Series, no. 1263 (Okinawa Japan: Elsevier, 2003): 791-794.

28. Hoyle, pp. 168-69; David M. Vu, Alberdina W. de Boer, Lisa Danzig, George Santos, Bridget Canty, Betty M. Flores, Dan M. Granoff, "Priming for Immunologic Memory in Adults by Meningococcal Group C Conjugate Vaccine," *Clinical and Vaccine Immunology* 13, no. 6 (June 2006): 605-10.

29. Hoyle, 159-169.

30. Interview with Michael A.W. Hattwick, M.D., Chief, Respiratory and Special Pathogens Branch, Viral Diseases Division, Bureau of Epidemiology, Center for Disease Control, Atlanta, Georgia, March 24, 1975.

31. Ibid., 159-69.

32. Charles Nicolle and C. Lebailly, *Compt. Rend. Acad. Sci.*, (1918) clxvii, 607; H.G. Gibson, F.B. Bowman, and J.L Connor, *British Medical Journal* (1918) ii, 645.

33. Wilson Smith, C.H. Andrews, and Patrick Playfair Laidlaw, "A Virus Obtained from Influenza Patients." *Lancet* 225, 8 July 1933, 66-68.

34. "A Revised System of Nomenclature for Influenza Viruses," *Bulletin of the World Health Organization* 45, no. 1 (1971): 119-24.

35. Ibid.

36. Edwin D. Kilbourne, "Flu to the Starboard! Man the Harpoons! Fill 'em with vaccine! Get the Captain! Hurry!" *New York Times*, 13 February 1976; Walter R. Dowdle, "Influenza Pandemic Periodicity, Virus Recycling, and the Art of Risk Assessment," *Emerging Infectuous Diseases* 12, no. 1 (January 2006): 34-39.

37. Gina Kolata, *Flu: The Story of the Great Influenza Pandemic of 1918 and the Search for the Virus that Caused It* (New York: Touchstone Press, 2001); *New Haven* (Conn.) *Journal Courier* 20 December 1977; 31 January 1978.

38. Dowdle, 2006.

39. Knight, 98.

40. Edwin D. Kilbourne, "A Virologist's Perspective on the 1918-

1919 Pandemic," in *The Spanish Influenza Pandemic of 1918-19: New Perspectives*, ed. Howard Phillips and David Killingray, (New York: Routledge, 2003), 32.

41. Ibid.

42. Knight, 95.

43. Dowdle, 2006.

44. David Thomson, and Robert Thomson, *Annals of the Pickett-Thomson Research Laboratory*, vols. 9 and 10, monograph 16: *Influenza* (Baltimore: Williams & Wilkins, 1934), 4.

45. Ibid.

46. Gabriela Torrea, Viviane Chenal-Francisque, Alexandre Leclercq, Elisabeth Carniel, "Efficient Tracing of Global Isolates of *Yersinia pestis* by Restriction Fragment Length Polymorphism Analysis Using Three Insertion Sequences as Probes," *Journal of Clinical Microbiology* 44, no. 6 (June 2006): 2084-92.

47. See the original listing in John R. Mote, "Human and Swine Influenza," in *Virus and Rickettsial Diseases: With Especial Consideration of Their Public Health Significance*, [Harvard School of Public Health Symposium, 12-17 June 1939], (Cambridge: Harvard UP, 1940), 433.

48. Thomson and Thomson, vol. 1, p. 7.

49. Knight, 88.

50. Arthur Stanley, M.D., Health Officer, Shanghai Municipal Council, Public Health Report 1918, "Medical Reports," *China Medical Journal* 33 (1919): 273.

51. See Chap. 6, "Respiratory Diseases," in John Duffy, *Epidemics in Colonial America* (Baton Rouge: Louisiana State UP, 1953), 184-85.

52. Ibid., 186.

53. Ibid., 187.

54. Ibid., 187-88.

55. Ibid., 188.

56. Ibid.

57. Ibid., 189.

58. Knight, 89.

59. Wilson and Miles, 10-11.

60. *Reports of the Director of the Laboratories and the Director of the Hospital*, vol. 7, *Rockefeller Institute for Medical Research* (New York: Rockefeller University Archives, 1919), 60-62, 172-76.

61. War Department, *Annual Report of the Secretary of War for the Fiscal Year 1918*.

62. U.S. Department of the Army, *The Medical Department of the United States Army in the World War*, 61.

63. Edwin O. Jordan, *Epidemic Influenza: A Survey* (Chicago: American Medical Association, 1927), 64, 74-75.

64. Taubenberger, 2005.

65. Lone Simonsen, Matthew J. Clarke, Lawrence B. Schonberger, Nancy H. Arden, Nancy J. Cox, and Keiji Fukuda, "Pandemic Versus Epidemic Influenza Mortality: A Pattern of Changing Age Distribution," *Journal of Infectious Diseases* 178 (1998): 53-60.

66. Jordan., 47, 198.

67. In the fall of 1918 New York's Governor Whitman appointed a special Influenza Commission. At the second meeting, held on November 22, 1918, the chairman, State Commissioner of Health Hermann M. Biggs, M.D., noted that the "last great epidemic before '91 was in 1832. The age incidence was the same—young and old escaped, and young adults heavily affected. 1891-92 was the other way." Copies of the

minutes of the Influenza Commission can be found in the Papers of C.-E. A. Winslow, Series I, Box 12, which are listed under the Department of Public Health, Sterling Library, Yale University, New Haven.

68. Ministry of Health, United Kingdom, "The influenza epidemic in England and Wales, 1957-1958," in *Reports on Public Health and Medical Subjects* 100 (London: Ministry of Health), 1960; Jeffrey K. Taubenberger, Ann H. Reid, Thomas A. Janczewski, Thomas G. Fanning, "Integrating Historical, Clinical and Molecular Genetic Data in Order to Explain the Origin and Virulence of the 1918 Spanish Influenza Virus," *Philosophical Transactions of the Royal Society of London, Series B, Biological Sciences* 356, 29 December 2001, 1829-1839

69. Crosby, 317.

70. Thomson and Thomson, vol. 1, p. 771.

71. Katarzyna Rybicka and Lidia B. Brydak, "Encephalopathy and Encephalitis – Influenza-Associated Neurological Sequels," *Polski Merkuriusz Lekarski* 19 (October 2005): 501-05; M.H. Smidt, H. Stroink, J.F. Bruinenberg, and M.F. Peeters, "Encephalopathy Associated with Influenza A," *European Journal of Paediatric Neurology* 8, no. 5 (2004): 257-60.

72. Tim Mears, "Acupuncture in the Treatment of Post Viral Fatigue Syndrome – a Case Report," *Acupuncture in Medicine* 23, no. 3 (September 2005): 141-45; Benjamin H. Natelson, Shelley A. Weaver, Chin-Lin Tseng, and John E. Ottenweller, "Spinal Fluid Abnormalities in Patients with Chronic

Fatigue Syndrome," *Clinical and Diagnostic Laboratory Immunology* 12, no. 1 (January 2005): 52-55.

73. See paper "Epidemic Encephalitis or Sleepy Sickness," written by Simon Flexner, for *Scientific American*, and dated September 1927, p. 1, *Papers of the Simon Flexner Library of the American Philosophical Society*, Philadelphia.

74. Ibid., 3.

75. Ibid.

76. See paper "Epidemic Encephalitis"—Remarks by Dr. Simon Flexner before the Annual Conference of Health Officers and Public Health Nurses held at Saratoga, New York, June 24, 1924, *Flexner Papers*.

77. "Epidemic Encephalitis or Sleepy Sickness," p. 4, *Flexner Papers*.

78. Rybicka & Brydak, 2005.

79. "Epidemic Encephalitis," pp. 6-10, *Flexner Papers*. He came to this conclusion even though he knew that the lungs of some of the fatal cases showed a bronchopneumonia along with the brain inflammation.

80. Eugenia T. Gamboa, Abner Wolf, Melvin D. Yahr, Donald H. Harter, Philip E. Duffy, Herbert Barden, and Konrad C. Hsu, "Influenza Virus Antigen in Postencephalitic Parkinsonian Brain: Detection by Immunofluorescence," *Archives of Neurology* 31, no. 4 (October 1974): 228-32.

81. Sherman McCall, James M. Henry, Ann H. Reid, and Jeffrey K. Taubenberger, "Influenza RNA Not Detected in Archival Brain Tissues from Acute Encephalitis Lethargica Cases or in Postencephalitic Parkinson Cases," *Journal of Neuropathology and Experimental*

Pathology, 60, no. 7 (July 2001): 696-704.; K.C. Lo, Jennian F. Geddes, Rod S. Daniels, and John S. Oxford, "Lack of Detection of Influenza Genes in Archived Formalin-fixed, Paraffin Wax-embedded Brain Samples of Encephalitis Lethargica Patients from 1916 to 1920," *Virchows Archiv* 442, no. 6 (June 2003): 591-96.

82. B.C. Easterly, 2003. "Swine Influenza: Historical Perspectives." *Proceedings of the 4th International Symposium on Emerging and Re-emerging Pig Diseases,* Rome, Italy, 29 June – 2 July, 2003: pp. 241-44.

83. William Arthur Hagan and Dorsey William Bruner, *Infectious Diseases of Domestic Animals: With Special Reference to Etiology, Diagnosis, and Biologic Therapy,* 3rd ed. (Ithaca, New York: Comstock, 1957), 862-63.

84. Thomson and Thomson, vol. 2, 629-34.

85. Robert C. Easterday, "Influenza," in *Diseases Transmitted From Animals to Man,* ed. William T. Hubbert, William F. McCulloch, Paul R. Schnurrenberger and Thomas G. Hull, 6th ed. (Springfield, Ill.: Charles C. Thomas, 1975), 839.

86. Ibid.

87. "Sources of Influenza," *British Medical Journal,* 30 June 1973, pp. 730-33.

88. Christopher Andrewes, Patrick P. Laidlaw, and Wilson Smith, "Influenza: Observations on the Recovery of Virus from Man and on the Antibody Content of Human Sera," *British Journal of Experimental Pathology* 17 (1935), 579-581

89. Sources of Influenza, 730-33.

90. Taubenberger, et al. (2005), Sources of Influenza, 730-33

91. Sources of Influenza, 730-33.

92. Sources of Information, 730-33.

93. See Wilson and Miles, vol. 2, "Secondary Bronchopneumonia," pp. 2016-17.

94. U.S. Department of the Army, *The Medical Department of the United States Army in the World War,* 145-50.

CHAPTER 2: THE SILENT FOE (SPRING 1918)

1. John F. Fulton, *Harvey Cushing: A Biography* (Springfield, Ill.: Charles C. Thomas, Publishers, 1946), 228.

2. "The Reminiscences of Dr. Joseph Aub," Oral History Research Office, Columbia University, 1968, no. 366, 2 vols. pp. 150-52.

3. William R. Noyes, "Influenza Epidemic 1918-1919: A Misplaced Chapter in United States Social and Institutional History," Ph.D. dissertation, University of California, Los Angeles, 1968, p. 6.

4. Alfred W. Crosby, *America's Forgotten Pandemic: The Influenza of 1918,* 2d ed. (Cambridge: Cambridge UP, 2003), 17.

5. John M. Barry, *The Great Influenza: The Epic Story of the Deadliest Plague in History* (New York: Viking Penguin, 2004) 147-148.

6. See article written by the historian, Albert Bushnell Hart, "Baker and His Task," *New York Times,* 7 April 1918, magazine section, pp. 1-2.

7. *New York Times,* 20 January 1918.

8. Frederick Palmer, *Newton D. Baker: America at War,* 2 vols. (New York: Dodd, Mead & Co., 1931), 2: 54-79.

9. Victor C. Vaughan, *A Doctor's Memories* (Indianapolis: Bobbs-Merrill Co., 1926), 416-17.

10. Barry, 150.

11. Ibid., 137-139.

12. Ibid., 136.

13. *Washington Post*, 19 December 1917.

14. *New York Times*, 26 January 1918.

15. Ibid.

16. Ibid.

17. Ibid., 27 February 1918.

18. Ibid.

19. Item #118, January 4, 1918, Box 8, in MSS No. 9776, Papers of Newton D. Baker, Library of Congress.

20. *New York Times*, 24 February, 2 March 1918.

21. Vaughan, 422-31.

22. Ibid.

23. Ibid., 428-31.

24. Barry, 165-166.

25. Elliott Roosevelt, ed. *F. D. R.: His Personal Letters 1905-1928* (New York: Duell, Sloan & Pearce, 1948), 369-70.

26. Diary No. 13, March 11-April 24, 1918, Series II, MSS No. 466, Colonel E. M. House Collection, Yale Sterling Library, New Haven.

27. *New York Times*, 9 March 1918.

28. Ibid., 16 March 1918.

29. Ibid., 17 March 1918.

30. Ibid., 20 March 1918.

31. Ibid., 21 March 1918.

32. Ibid., 22 March 1918.

33. Ibid., 2 March 1918.

34. Ibid., 29 April 1918.

35. U.S. Department of the Navy, Bureau of Medicine and Surgery, *Annual Report of the Surgeon General: U.S. Navy* (1919) (Washington, D.C.: Government Printing Office, 1919), 369.

36. U.S. Department of Health, Education, and Welfare, Public Health Service, *Mortality From Influenza and Pneumonia in 50 Large Cities of the United States 1919-1929*, by Selwyn D. Collins, W. H. Frost, Mary Gover, and Edgar Sydenstricker, Reprint no. 1415 from *Public Health Reports* 45, 26 September 1930, p. 32 (Washington, D.C. Government Printing Office, 1930), p. 32.

37. Ibid. 27-43.

38. Ibid.

39. Ibid.

40. U.S. Department of the Navy, *Annual Report (1919)*, 367.

41. Ibid.

42. Ibid.

43. Ibid., 368.

44. Ibid., 368-69.

45. Edward Robb Ellis, *Echoes of Distant Thunder: Life in the United States 1914-1918* (New York: Coward, McCann & Geoghegan, 1975), 262.

46. Barry, 169, Crosby, 19 quoting Opie, E. et al., "Pneumonia at Camp Funston," *Journal of the American Medical Association*, 72 (January 1919): 114-115.

47. "Endemic Influenza," a paper read before the New York Clinical Society, January 27, 1922, pp. 14-15, Section I, Papers of Rufus Ivory Cole, Library of the American Philosophical Society, Philadelphia.

48. Letter to "DDB," February 19, 1918, Papers of Francis Gilman Blake, M.D., in possession of Dr. John B. Blake, Bethesda, Maryland.

49. Ibid., 26 March 1918.

50. *Washington Post*, 22 January 1918.

51. "Endemic Influenza," Cole papers.

52. U.S. Department of the Army, *The Medical Department in the World War*, pp. 78, 83, 133, 135-36.

53. Ibid.

54. Ibid., 23.

55. *North China Herald and Supreme Court and Consular Gazette* (Shanghai), 8

June 1918.

56. Robert Frost and Elinor Frost, *Family Letters of Robert and Elinor Frost*, ed. Arnold E. Grade. Albany: State University of New York Press, 1972): 27-28.

57. *New York Times*, 6 April 1918.

58. Leonard Keene Hirshberg, "The Spanish Influenza," *Munsey's Magazine* 65 (January 1919): 664-68.

59. Cushing, 466.

60. Crosby, 26; Edwin O. Jordan, *Epidemic Influenza: A Survey* (Chicago: American Medical Association, 1927), 83.

61. Jordan, 70-75.

62. Charles C. Gill, "Overseas Transportation of the United States Troops," *Current History* 9 (1918-1919): 411. (These figures are somewhat higher than those issued in the *Reports of the Commander-in-Chief, A.E.F.*, 1948. Evidently the Gill figures include civilians who accompanied the A.E.F.)

63. U.S. Department of Labor, *Annual Report of the Commissioner General of Immigration to the Secretary of Labor*, Fiscal Year ended June 30, 1922 (Washington, D.C.: Government Printing Office, 1922), p. 142.

64. *Washington Post*, 25 December 1917.

65. Ibid., 6 January 1918.

66. Ibid., 13 January 1918.

67. Ibid., 16 January 1918.

68. *North China Herald* (Shanghai), 12 January 1918.

69. See reports of disagreement over the diagnosis of pneumonic plague in the *China Weekly Review* (Shanghai), 19 January 1918, and in the *North China Herald* (Shanghai), 19 January 1918.

70. *North China Herald* (Shanghai), 19 January 1918.

71. Ibid.

72. Ibid., 30 March 1918.

73. Ibid., 23 March 1918.

74. Ibid., 30 March 1918.

75. *China Weekly Review* (Shanghai), 20 April 1918.

76. S. T. Lee, [Paris, France], "Some of the different Aspects Between Influenza, Pneumonia, and Pneumonic Plague," *New York Medical Journal* 110 (September 6, 1919): 401-03.

77. U.S. Department of Labor, *Annual Report of the Commissioner General on Immigration to the Secretary of Labor*, Fiscal Year ended June 30, 1922 (Washington, D.C.: Government Printing Office, 1922), p. 142. See Judith Blick, "The Chinese Labor Camps in World War I," *Papers on China*, vol. 9, from the East Asia Regional Studies Seminar, Harvard University, August 1955, p. 120; U.S. Department of Labor, Bureau of Labor Statistics, *Chinese Migrations, With Special Reference to Labor Conditions. Bulletin of the U.S. Bureau of Labor Statistics*, no. 340 (Washington, D.C.: Government Printing Office, 1923), p. 143; and Daryl Klein, *With the Chinks* (London: John Lane, 1919), pp. 18, 28.

78. Blick, 114.

79. Klein, 56.

80. Klein, 56.

81. Klein, 56.

82. Ibid., 76.

83. Ibid., 61.

84. *North China Herald* (Shanghai), 9 February 1918.

85. See Klein. For a discussion of a visit in New York City, see p. 242.

86. From an interview with Ira Vaughan Hiscock, Professor of Public Health, Emeritus, Yale University,

August 15, 1975.

87. Helen Dore Boylston, *"Sister": The War Diary of a Nurse* (New York: Ives Washburn, 1927), 7.

88. U.S. Department of the Army, Historical Division, *United States Army in the World War 1917-1919*, Reports of the Commander-in-Chief, A.E.F., Staff Sections and Services (Washington, D.C.: Government Printing Office, 1948), p. 370.

89. Boylston, 82-83.

90. *New York Times*, 28, 29 April 1918.

91. Ibid., 1 June 1918.

92. Ibid., 7 June 1918.

93. Rudolf Binding, *A Fatalist at War*, trans. by Ian F. D. Morrow (Boston: Houghton Mifflin, 1929), 241.

94. *New York Times*, 21 June 1918.

95. Ibid., 22 June 1918.

96. Ibid., 27 June 1918.

97. Ibid.

98. Barry, 178-179

99. *New York Times*, 3 July 1918.

100. Ibid., 9 July 1918.

101. Ibid

102. Ibid., 11 July 1918.

103. Ibid., 13 July 1918.

104. Ibid., 14 July 1918.

105. Ibid., 26 July 1918.

CHAPTER 3: A KIND OF PLAGUE (FALL 1918)

1. Francis Gilman Blake to "DDB," October 21, 1918, Papers of Francis Gilman Blake, M.D. in the possession of Dr. John B. Blake, Bethesda, Maryland. Hereafter all Blake notations refer to letters from Francis G. Blake to "DDB."

2. Diary of the Hong Kong Visit, 1918, Correspondence, Papers of Peter K. Olitsky, M.D., Library of the American Philosophical Society, Philadelphia.

3. James Kerney to Joseph P. Tumulty, August 7, 1918, Container J., *Papers of Joseph P. Tumulty*, Library of Congress.

4. John F. Fulton, *Harvey Cushing: A Biography* (Springfield, Ill.: Charles C. Thomas, Publishers, 1946), 413.

5. Ibid., 418.

6. Ibid., 427.

7. Rudolf Binding, *A Fatalist at War*, trans. by Ian F. D. Morrow (Boston: Houghton Mifflin, 1929), 241.

8. Ibid.

9. U.S. Department of the Army, *United States Army in the World War*, p. 372.

10. *New York Times*, 18 August 1918; and George A. Soper, "The Pandemic in the Army Camps," *J.A.M.A.* 71 (1918): 1907.

11. Soper, Ibid.

12. John Dos Passos, *The Fourteenth Chronicle: Letters and Diaries of John Dos Passos*, ed. Townsend Ludington (Boston: Gambit, 1973), 207.

13. John Dos Passos, *Nineteen Nineteen* (Boston: Houghton Mifflin, 1932, Signet Classic, New American Library Edition, 1969), 34.

14. "Brief Outline of Activities of the Public Health Service in Combating the Influenza Epidemic 1918-1919," General Records of the Public Health Service, General Files 1897-1923, No. 1622, Record Group 90, *National Archives*, Washington, D.C.

15. Ibid.

16. *New York Times*, 16 August 1918.

17. Ibid., 17 August 1918.

18. Ibid., 18, 19 August , 5 September 1918.

19. *The Red Cross Bulletin* 2, 5 August 1918, p. 2.

20. *New York Times*, 19 August 1918.

21. U.S. Department of the Army, *The Medical Department in the World War*, p. 78.

22. "Oral History Transcript," interview by Saul Benison, p. 14, Box 1, Papers of Peter K. Olitsky, *M.D.*, *Rockefeller University Archives*, New York, N.Y.: and Saul Benison, prep., *Tom Rivers: Reflections on a Life in Medicine and Science: An Oral History Memoir* (Cambridge: MIT Press, 1967), 320.

23. Cushing, 276-77.

24. Ibid., p. 302; Hugh Young, *Hugh Young: A Surgeon's Autobiography* (New York Harcourt, Brace, 1940), 387.

25. 23 July 1918, Blake Papers.

26. Ibid., 30 July 1918.

27. Ibid., 2 August 1918.

28. Ibid., 8 August 1918.

29. Ibid., 9 August 1918.

30. Ibid., 16 August 1918.

31. Ibid., 17 August 1918.

32. Ibid., 30 August 1918.

33. Ibid., 12 September 1918.

34. Ibid.

35. Simon Flexner and James Thomas Flexner, *William Henry Welch and the Heroic Age of American Medicine* (New York: Viking Press, 1941): 372.

36. "Remarks as Toastmaster at the 50th Reunion of Yale '70," p. 11, Subject Index "World War"—War Service, Papers of William H. Welch, M.D., William Welch Library, Baltimore.

37. According to V.C. Vaughn (*A Doctor's Memories*, 1926), the tour of the Southern States took place in August. However, Dr. William. H. Welch kept a diary of the trip, Diary #12, dated September 4-21, 1918, which may be found in his Papers.

38. Vaughn, *A Doctor's Memories*, p. 431. However, according to the *Reports of the Director of the Laboratories and the Director of the Hospital*, vol. 6, October 1918, p. 346, Rockefeller University Archives, New York, N.Y., the camps involved were Camp Jackson and Camp Dix. Perhaps all four camps were in the program.

39. U.S. Department of the Navy, *Annual Report (1919)*, p. 371; and Soper, 1900.

40. "Girls of Boston Must Cut Out That Germy Kiss," unidentified clipping, Records of the Bureau of Medicine and Surgery. Record Group 52, File 126976 (1918), *National Archives*, Washington, D.C.

41. U.S. Department of the Navy, *Annual Report (1919)*, p. 446.

42. Robert Frost and Elinor Frost, *Family Letters of Robert and Elinor Frost*, ed. Arnold E. Grade. Albany: State University of New York Press, 1972): 30-31. [Hereafter referred to as Grade.]

43. P.M. Ashburn "*A History of the Medical Department of the United States Army*" (Boston: Houghton Mifflin, 1929): 318.

44. "The Etiology and Prevention of Influenza," pp. 3-4, Category I, Papers of Rufus Ivory Cole, Library of the American Philosophical Society, Philadelphia.

45. Crosby, 9.

46. Ibid.

47. Soper, 1900. [The table as printed in the *Journal of the American Medical Association* shows an equal number of cases of influenza and pneumonia—571—in the period of slow decline. This could possibly be a printing error.]

48. Ibid.

49. John M. Barry, *The Great Influenza: The Epic Story of the Deadliest Plague in History* (New York: Viking Penguin, 2004) 191.

50. Soper, 1900.

51. Crosby, p.11 quoting Johns Hopkins University Institute of the History of Medicine, William Henry Welch Library, William Henry Welch Papers, Address delivered on the evening of December 27, 1919, at the New Century Club before the Committee of Twenty and invited guests of Utica, New York, pp 8-10, 14.

52. Carla Morrissey, "Influenza, 1918," Arlington, Va.: PBS Home Video, 1998.

53. Robert St. John, *This Was My World* (Garden City, NY: Doubleday, 1953), 49-50.

54. Ibid.

55. Peter D. Olch, prep., "Autobiographical Memoir of Shields Warren," Oral History, 1973, pp. 9-10, History of Medicine Division, *National Library of Medicine*, Bethesda, Maryland.

56. Ibid.

57. *Washington Post*, 13 October 1918.

58. Soper, 1904.

59. 22 September 1918, Blake Papers.

60. Ibid.

61. Ibid.

62. Ibid., 24 September 1918.

63. Ibid., 25 September 1918.

64. Ibid., 2 October 1918.

65. Ibid., 4-6 October 1918.

66. Ibid.

67. Ibid., 12-16 October 1918.

68. "The Reminiscences of Dana W. Atchley, M.D.," Oral History Research Office, Columbia University, 1964, No. 545 I-B, pp. 94-95.

69. "The Reminiscences of A. R. Dochez, M.D.," Oral History Research Office, Columbia University, 1957, No. 267 I-A, pp. 73-77.

70. Ibid.

71. Ibid.

72. "Reminiscences of Dana W. Atchley, M.D.," pp. 94-95.

73. Grade, 31-33.

74. Ibid.

75. Ibid.

76. Brief Outline of Activities of the Public Health Service."

77. *New York Times*, 22 September 1918.

78. W.A. Bolton to the President, San Diego, Calif., September 26, 1918, Container 210, Papers of William Gibbs McAdoo, *Library of Congress.*

79. *Washington Post*, 8 October 1918.

80. *Washington Post*, 22 September 1918.

81. *Washington Post*, 25 September 1918.

82. *Washington Post*, 28 September 1918.

83. The Henry Lewis Stimson Diaries 1909-1928, vols. 1-8, pp. 76-77, Yale Sterling Library, *Yale University*, New Haven.

84. "The Mobilization of the American National Red Cross during the Influenza Pandemic 1918," Library of the American National Red Cross, Washington, D.C.

85. "Brief Outline of Activities of the Public Health Service," p. 2.

86. *New York Times*, 26 September 1918.

87. *Washington Post*, 27 September 1918.

88. "The Mobilization of the

American National Red Cross during the Influenza Pandemic 1918–1919. 1920. Geneva, Switzerland, p. 24.

89. *Washington Post*, 28 September 1918.

90. *New York Times*, 29 September 1918.

91. "Brief Outline of Activities of the Public Health Service," p. 3.

92. "The Mobilization of the American National Red Cross."

93. Permelia Murnan Doty, "A Retrospect of the Influenza Epidemic," *Public Health Nurse* 11, no 12 (1919): 949-57.

94. Ibid.

95. Doty, 1919; Edna L. Foley, "Department of Public Health Nursing in Charge of Edna L Foley," *American Journal of Nursing* 19, no. 3 (1918): 189-95.

96. Mary E. Westphal, "Influenza Vignettes," *Public Health Nurse* 11, no. 2 (1919): 129-33.

97. Foley, 1918.

98. *Washington Post*, 1, 2 October 1918.

99. Treasury Department Memo, 2 October 1918, Container 211, #328, Papers of William Gibbs McAdoo, *Library of Congress*

100. Ibid., 3 October 1918.

101. Ibid., 4 October 1918.

102. *Washington Post*, 2 October 1918.

103. Ibid.

104. Ibid., 3 October 1918.

105. Ibid., 4 October 1918.

106. Eva Le Gallienne, *At 33* (New York: Longmans, Green, 1934): 139-41.

107. *Washington Post*, 3-7 October 1918.

108. Katherine Anne Porter, "Pale Horse Pale Rider," in Collected Stories of Katherine Anne Porter (New York: Harcourt, Brace & World, New American Library, A Plume Book, 1970): 299.

109. *Washington Post*, 12 October 1918.

110. Ibid., 21 November 1918.

111. Ibid., 13 October 1918.

112. Ibid., 12 October 1918.

113. Ibid., 13 October 1918.

114. Ibid., 18 October 1918.

115. Ibid., 10 October 1918.

116. *New Haven* (Conn.) *Union*, 30 October 1918.

117. Ibid.

118. Ibid.

119. *Washington Post*, 13 October 1918.

120. Ibid., 14-15 October 1918.

121. C. E. Winslow and J. F. Rogers, "Statistics of the 1918 Epidemic of Influenza in Connecticut," *Journal of Infectious Diseases*. 26 (1920): 185-216.

122. *Washington Post*, 16 October 1918.

123. Crosby, 82.

124. Harriet Hasty Ferrel, "Influenza, 1918," PBS HomeVideo, 1998.

125. Crosby, 83.

126. Ibid., 18 November 18, 1918.

127. Ibid., 18 November 1918.

128. Palmer, *Newton D. Baker*, 365.

129. Ibid.

130. Ibid., 366.

131. Crosby, 137.

132. [Vice-Admiral] Albert Gleaves [USN], *A History of the Transport Service: Adventures and Experiences of U.S. Transports and Cruisers in the World War* (New York: George H. Doran, 1921): 190-91.

133. Ibid.

134. U.S. Department of the Navy, *Annual Report (1919)*, p. 66.

135. Crosby, 137.

136. Ibid., 38.

137. Cromwell, B. and Wilson, R.F. *How America Went to War. The Road to France* (New Haven: Yale UP, 1921), vol. 2, pp. 442-43.

138. Cushing, 472-73.

139. U.S. Department of the Army, *The Medical Department in the World War*, pp. 127-29.

140. U.S. Department of the Army, *United States Army in the World War*, p. 373.

141. James M. Howard to Mrs. Howard, 20 November 1918, Box I, General Correspondence, MSS no. 471, Papers of James M. Howard, Yale Sterling Library, Yale university, New Haven.

142. *Washington Post*, 12, 22 October 1918.

143. Ibid., 6 November 1918.

144. An Account of the Influenza Epidemic in Perry County, Kentucky. 1919. 8/14/19, RG 200, Box 689, *National Archives*; John M. Barry, 1918 Revisited: Lessons and Suggestions for Further Inquiry in *"The Threat of Pandemic Influenza Are we Ready?"* Workshop Summary. Ed. S.L. Knobler (Washington D.C., The National Academies Press, 2005): 66.

145. Grade, 35-37.

146. *Washington Post*, 23 October 1918.

147. *New York Times*, 20, 25 October 1918.

148. Ibid., 29 October 1918.

149. October 26, 1918, Blake Papers.

CHAPTER 4: ONE WAR ENDS

1. According to the minutes of the Influenza Commission, #2, November 22, 1918, C.E.A. Winslow, Series I, Box 12, Department of Public Health Papers, Yale Sterling Library, Yale University, New Haven, four Hopkins nurses died during the fall of 1918. Yet, according to James A. Douall and Anne M. Bahlke, in their article "Epidemic Influenza: A Comparison of Clinical Observations in a Major and a Minor Epidemic," *American Journal of Hygiene* 17 (1933): 562-80, only three Hopkins nurses died that fall.

2. William H. Welch to F. C. Walcott, October 16 and 23, 1918, Correspondence 1918, Frederic Collin Walcott Correspondence and Manuscripts, Yale Sterling Library, Yale University, New Haven. Walcott was Welch's nephew.

3. Lucy M. Smith to Woodrow Wilson, October 23, 1918, Presidential Papers Microfilm, Series 2, Reel 101, Woodrow Wilson Papers.

4. Diary kept by Head Usher 1913-1921, 1918, Presidential Papers Microfilm, Series 2, Reel 3, Woodrow Wilson Papers.

5. T. R. Marshall to N. D. Baker, October 31, 1918, Container 7, June-December 1918, M., Papers of Newton D. Baker, Library of Congress.

6. Douglas Fairbanks to Joseph Tumulty and Woodrow Wilson to Joseph Tumulty, October 29, 1918, Container 5, Woodrow Wilson, Papers of Joseph P. Tumulty, Library of Congress.

7. *Washington Post*, 20 October 1918.

8. *New York Times*, 9, 11 September 1918.

9. Ibid., 12 September 1918.

10. Diaries, No. 14, September 13, 1918, Colonel E. M. House Collection. Yale Sterling Library, Yale University, New Haven.

11. *Billboard*, 5 October 1918.

12. Ibid.

13. Ibid.

14. Ibid., 19 October 1918.

15. *New York Times*, 13 October 1918, section 4, p. 4.

16. Hollis Alpert, *The Barrymores* (New York: The Dial Press, 1964): 188, 192.

17. Ibid.

18. *Billboard*, 19 October 1918.

19. Ibid., and 9 November 1918.

20. Ibid., 9 November 1918.

21. Ibid., 16, 30 November, 7 December 1918.

22. Ibid., 7, 14, 21 December 1918.

23. R. Carlyle Buley, *The American Life Convention 1906-1952: A Study in the History of Life Insurance*. 2 vols. (New York: Appleton-Century-Crofts, 1953): 538.

24. Ibid., 488-89.

25. Marquis James, *The Metropolitan Life: A Study in Business Growth* (New York: Viking Press, 1947): 204.

26. *Washington Post*, 5 December 1918.

27. Earl Chapin May and Will Oursler, *The Prudential: A Story of Human Security* (Garden City, N.Y.: Doubleday & Co., 1950): 179-83.

28. James, 205.

29. Buley, 538.

30. Ibid., 560-61.

31. May and Oursler, 180-81.

32. "Alcoholic Drinks as a Preventative of 'Influenza,' an Erroneous Impression," J.A. Nydegger,

Surgeon, 11 October 1918, no. 1622, Bureau of the Public Health Service, Record Group 12, *National Archives*, Washington, D.C.

33. Telegram to Blue, U.S.P.H.S. Service, from Spartanburg, South Carolina, 6 December 1918, no. 1622, General Files 1897-1923, Bureau of the Public Health Service, Record Group 90, *National Archives*, Washington, D.C.

34. R. Blue to Ward, Spartanburg, South Carolina, 9 December 1918, no. 1622, General Files 1897-1923, Bureau of the Public Health Service, R. G. 90, National Archives, Washington, D.C.

35. *Washington Post*, 11 February 1919.

36. Cortez Ewing, *Congressional Elections 1896-1944: The Sectional Basis of Political Democracy in the House of Representatives*. (Norman: U of Oklahoma Press, 1947): 35.

37. Treasury Department Telegram to S. R. Bertron, November 4, 1918, Container 22, Papers of William Gibbs McAdoo, *Library of Congress*

38. Thomas L. Sidlo to Newton D. Baker, November 7, 1918, Container 7, N. D. Baker Papers.

39. Ibid.

40. Blanche W. Jacobi to Newton D. Baker, October 30, 1918, Box 14, #452, N. D. Baker Papers..

41. Newton D. Baker to Brand Whitlock, November 2, 1918, Box 8, #173, N. D. Baker Papers.

42. Ibid.

43. John F. Fulton, *Harvey Cushing: A Biography* (Springfield, Ill.: Charles C. Thomas, 1946): 490.

44. Ibid., 492-93.

45. Ibid., 495.

46. Diary No. 14, November 11, 1918, Colonel E. M. House Collection; Florence Jaffray Hurst Harriman, *From Pinafores to Politics* (New York: Henry Holt & Co., 1923): 297.

47. M.A. DeWolfe Howe, *John Jay Chapman and His Letters* (Boston: Houghton Mifflin, 1937): 334-37.

48. Robert Frost, *The Letters of Robert Frost to Louis Untermeyer.* Edited by Louis Untermeyer (New York: Holt, Rinehart and Winston, 1963): 77.

49. Ibid.

50. Robert Frost, *Selected Letters of Robert Frost.* Edited by Lawrence Thompson (New York: Holt, Rinehart and Winston, 1964): 233.

51. Harriman, 296.

52. William Wordsworth, *The Prelude or Growth of a Poet's Mind* (Text of 1905), ed. Ernest de Selincourt (London: Oxford UP, 1964): 196.

53. Boylston, 173.

54. Ibid., 168-69.

55. Loyal Davis, *A Surgeon's Odyssey* (New York: Doubleday & Co., 1973): 74-75.

56. Ibid.

57. Frances Parkinson Keyes, *All Flags Flying: Reminiscences of Frances Parkinson Keyes* (New York: McGraw-Hill, 1972): 124.

58. Ibid., 124-26.

59. Ibid.

60. Frederic Collin Walcott to W. S. Walcott, January 4, 1919, Walcott Correspondence and Manuscripts.

61. Thomas M. Carothers to William G. McAdoo, December 9, 1918, McAdoo Papers.

62. Mrs. Edw. Stotesbury to Hon. Josephus Daniels, telegram dated 15 October 1918, No. 127706, Bureau of Medicine and Surgery, Record Group 52, National Archives, Washington, D.C.

63. John W. Cavanagh to U.S. Navy Department, 19 October 1918, no. 127706, Bureau of Medicine and Surgery, R.G. 52.

64. Office of Medical Officer in Charge, U.S.P.H.S., West Point, Mississippi, to Surgeon General, U.S.P.H.S., Washington, D.C. 26 September 1918, no. 1622, Bureau of the Public Health Service, R.G. 12.

65. "Order from the Board of Health—Supplemental Rules."

66. Ibid.

67. Robert Oleson to Surgeon General, U.S.P.H.S., 11 December 1918, no. 1622, General Files 1897-1923, Bureau of the Public Health Service, R.G. 90.

68. General Letter no. 39, December 14, 1918, Entry E2-D4, Council of National Defense, R.G. 62, National Archives, Washington, D.C.

69. 18 November 1918, Blake papers.

70. Ibid., 21 November 1918.

71. Ibid., 28 November 1918.

72. Ibid., 11 December 1918.

73. Ibid., 15, 17 December 1918.

74. Eugene Lindsay Opie, Allen W. Freeman, Francis G. Blake, James C. Small, Thomas M. Rivers, *Journal of the American Medical Association*, 11 January and 22 February 1919.

75. Milton Joseph Rosenau, *Journal of the American Medical Association*, 2 August 1919; Gina Kolata, *Flu The Story of the Great Influenza Pandemic of 1918 and the Search for the Virus That Caused It* (New

York, Touchstone, 2001): 55.

76. *Washington Post*, 17 November, 10 December 1918; *New York Times*, 22 December 1918.

77. *Washington Post*, 21, 22 December 1918, 1 January 1919.

78. *New York Times*, 12 November 1918.

79. Ibid., 4 December 1918.

80. John Dos Passos, *The Fourteenth Chronicle: Letters and Diaries of John Dos Passos*, ed. Townsend Ludington (Boston: Gambit, 1973), 211-25.

81. Ibid., 226.

82. Ibid., 232.

83. *New York Times*, 17 December 1918.

84. Ibid., 9 November 1918.

85. Ibid.

86. Ibid., 15 December 1918.

87. Ibid., 15, 16 December 1918.

88. Letter to Miss Marjorie Perry dated October 17, 1918, found under "Influenza," New England Division, no. 803.6, Library of the American National Red Cross, Washington, D.C.

89. Ibid.

90. Edwin O. Jordan, *Epidemic Influenza: A Survey* (Chicago: American Medical Association, 1927), 14, 272.

CHAPTER 5: "THE PARIS COLD"

1. Michael Corday, *The Paris Front: An Unpublished Diary 1914-1918* (New York: E. P. Dutton, 1934): 383.

2. Robert Frost. *The Letters of Robert Frost to Louis Untermeyer*. Edited by Louis Untermeyer (New York: Holt, Rinehart and Winston, 1963): 79.

3. Ibid.

4. See Richard Collier, *The Plague of the Spanish Lady: The Influenza Pandemic*

of 1918-1919 (New York: Atheneum, 1974): 287, and A. A. Hoehling, *The Great Epidemic* (Boston: Little, Brown, 1961): 9-10. Perhaps the writers took Dr. Rufus I. Cole too literally when he wrote that the epidemic "lasted, at least in its intensity, only for a short time and then disappeared as rapidly and mysteriously as it came." This statement is from a paper titled, "Endemic Influenza," that Cole read before the New York Clinical Society, January 27, 1922. It may be found in the Papers of Rufus Ivory Cole, Library of the American Philosophical Society, Philadelphia. Later statistical studies showed that the second wave of the epidemic lasted for thirty-one weeks.

5. "The Epidemic in Shansi: Pneumonic Plague or Influenza?" *China Medical Journal* 33 (1919): 169-73.

6. *New York Times*, 19 February 1919. However, it must be noted that 300 people died each day at the peak of the autumn wave of influenza.

7. Ibid., 15, 22 February, 1 March 1919.

8. *Washington Post*, 17 October 1918.

9. *New York Times*, 26 January 1919.

10. *Washington Post*, 20 October 1918, 10 January 1919; *New York Times*, 9 November 1918, 19 January 1919.

11. *New York Times*, 27, 28 December 1918; *Washington Post*, 4, 24 January 1919.

12. Minutes of the Fourth Meeting of The Governor's Influenza Commission Held at the Academy of Medicine, 14 February 1919, in C. -E.A. Winslow Papers, Department of Public Health. Manuscripts and Archives, Yale University Library, New Haven.

13. *New York Times*, 30 March 1919.

14. *Washington Post*, 27 January 1919.

15. *Billboard*, 25 January, 22 February, and 1 March 1919.

16. William G.B. Carson, *Dear Josephine: The Theatrical Career of Josephine Hull* (Norman: U of Oklahoma Press, 1965): 143-53.

17. Donald Richberg, *My Hero: The Indiscreet Memoirs of an Eventful but Unheroic Life: An Autobiography*. (New York: G. P. Putnam's Sons, 1954): 99.

18. *New York Times*, 5 January, 27 April 1919.

19. Ibid., 6 March 1919.

20. Ibid., 17 March 1919.

21. Ibid., 27 March 1919.

22. Diary for 1918, pp. 10-26, Diaries 1902-1940, Papers of Raymond Pearl, Library of the American Philosophical Society, Philadelphia.

23. Ibid.

24. Ibid., 6 November 1918.

25. Ibid., 7-9 November 1918.

26. Ibid., 10-11 November 1918.

27. Joseph C. Grew, *Turbulent Era: A Diplomatic Record of Forty Years 1904-1945*. Edited by Walter Johnson. (Boston: Houghton-Mifflin, 1952): 335; Diaries, 22 October 1918, Colonel E.M. House Collection, Yale Sterling Library, New Haven.

28. Diaries, Box 55, Folder 84, October 26-28, 1918, Papers of Gordon Auchincloss, Yale Sterling Library, New Haven.

29. Ibid., 11 November 1918.

30. Ibid.

31. Lawrence E. Gelfand, *The Inquiry: American Preparations for Peace 1917-1919* (New Haven: Yale UP, 1963): 165.

32. Johnson, Turbulent Era, pp. 356-57; Diaries, 15 November 1918, Auchincloss Papers.

33. Diaries, 18 November 1918, Auchinclose Papers.

34. Ibid., 19 November 1918.

35. Ibid., 20 November 1918.

36. Ibid., 21 November 1918.

37. Ibid., 23 November 1918.

38. Ibid.

39. Cable no. 165, November 25, 1918, Box 214, Colonel E. M. House Collection.

40. Diaries, November 30, 1918, Colonel E. M. House Collection.

41. Diaries, 1 December 1918, Auchinclose Papers.

42. Cable no. 209, 1 December 1918, Box 214, Colonel E. M. House Collection; Florence Jaffray Hurst Harriman, *From Pinafores to Politics* (New York: Henry Holt & Co., 1923): 297-300.

43. *New York American*, 23 November 1918.

44. Henry Wickham Steed, *Through Thirty Years 1892-1922: A Personal Narrative*. 2 vols. (Garden City, N.Y.: Doubleday, Page, 1924), vol. 2, p. 266.

45. Gelfand, 168-69.

46. "Letters From the Paris Peace Conference," 6 December 1918, Series I, Folder 136, Box 44, Charles Seymour Papers, MS No. 441, Yale Sterling Library, Yale University, New Haven; "Diary of Trip to Europe," December 7, 1918, Series III, Box 3, Correspondence 1918-1919, Clive Day Papers, MS No. 173, Yale Sterling Library, Yale University, New Haven.

47. The movie is mentioned in "Raymond B. Fosdick's Diary, 4-14 December 1918," p. 3, a copy of which

may be found in Series III, Folder 420, Box 283, Colonel E. M. House Collection. On Wilson's health, see Cary Grayson to Joseph P. Tumulty, December 12, 1918, *Papers of Joseph P. Tumulty*, Library of Congress.

48. Gelfand, 176-79; Charles Seymour, *Woodrow Wilson and the World War: A Chronicle of Our Own Times* (New Haven: Yale UP, 1921), Vol. 48 in *The Chronicles of America Series*, pp. 256-57; and Beatrice Bishop Berle and Travis Beal Jacobs, *Navigating the Rapids 1918-1971: From the Papers of Adolf A. Berle* (New York: Harcourt-Brace-Jovanovich, 1973): 7-11.

49. Johnson, *Turbulent Era*, pp. 388-89; Gelfand, p. 176: Seymour, p. 259; Herbert Hoover, *The Ordeal of Woodrow Wilson* (New York: McGraw-Hill, 1958): 84-85.

50. Letters dated 25-26 December 1918, Correspondence 1918-1919, Day Papers; letters dated 20-29 December 1918, Seymour Papers.

51. Letter dated 29 December 1918, Day Papers.

52. Letter dated 5 January 1919, Seymour Papers.

53. Letter dated 16 January 1919, Day Papers.

54. Letter dated 20 January 1919, Day Papers.

55. Diaries, 11-12 January 1919, Folder 87, Auchincloss Papers.

56. Diaries, 21 January 1919, Colonel E. M. House Collection.

57. Ibid.

58. Ibid., 26 January 1919.

59. *New York Telegram*, 14 January 1919.

60. Louisville (Kentucky) *Courier Journal*, 18 January 1919.

61. Washington, D.C., *Evening Star*, 22 January 1919.

62. Diaries, 22 January 1919, Auchincloss Papers. Actually, Miller had arrived in late 1918.

63. Ibid., 27 January 1919.

64. "Diaries of Vance C. McCormick, Member of the American War Mission to Inter-Allied Conference in London and Paris in 1917; and Advisor to President Wilson at the Peace Conference in Paris 1919," January 28-February 2, 1919, Box No. 15, Folder 2, Vance C. McCormick Papers, Yale Sterling Library, Yale University, New Haven.

65. Ibid., 19 February 1919.

66. Diaries, 16 February 1919, Auchincloss Papers.

67. Ibid., 6 February 1919.

68. Letter dated 8 February 1919, Seymour Papers.

69. Ibid., 23 January, 8, 9 February 1919.

70. Letter dated 13 February 1919, Day Papers.

71. Letter dated 15 February 1919, Seymour Papers.

72. Crosby, 185.

73. Ibid., 24 February 1919.

74. J. Donald Duncan to Gordon Auchincloss, 28 February 1919, Box 53, Folder 31, Auchincloss Papers.

75. One observer of President Wilson's twitching was Henry Morgenthau, *All in a Lifetime* (Garden City, N.Y.: Doubleday, Page, 1922): 305.

76. Cary Grayson to Joseph Tumulty, 13 March 1919, Tumulty Papers.

77. Gene Smith, *When the Cheering Stopped: The Last Years of Woodrow Wilson* (New York: William Morrow, 1964): 47.

78. *New York Times*, 2 February 1919.

79. Smith, 47-49.

80. Edward A. Weinstein, "Woodrow Wilson's Neurological Illness," *Journal of American History* 57 (1970-71): 324-51; also see Arthur Walworth, *Woodrow Wilson*, 2 vols. (New York: Longmans, Green, 1958), *World Prophet* 2: 297.

81. John Dos Passos, *Mr. Wilson's War* (Garden City, N.Y.: Doubleday, 1962): 477. John A. Garraty had also suggested that Wilson's illness was a stroke in his brief biography of Wilson 1956. Even before Garraty, Irwin H. (Ike) Hoover, White House Chief Usher, suggested in his *Forty-Two Years in the White House* (1934), that Wilson changed in Paris. Hoover wrote: "He went to bed ostensibly with a cold. When he got on his feet again he was a different man.... one thing was certain: he was never the same after this little spell of sickness."

82. Smith, 105-6.

83. Diaries, 3 April 1919, McCormick Papers.

84. Cary Grayson to Joseph Tumulty, cablegrams dated 4, 6, 8 April 1919, Tumulty Papers.

85. Ibid., 10 April 1919.

86. Lloyd George, *Memoirs of the Peace Conference*, (New Haven: Yale UP, 1939) vol. 1, 151, 185, 280; Hoover, Herbert, *America's First Crusade* (New York: Charles Scribner's Sons, 1942): 1, 40-41, 64; Crosby, 192-193.

87. Lincoln Steffens, *The Letters of Lincoln Steffens*. Edited by Ella Winter and Granville Hicks. 2 vols. (New York: Harcourt, Brace, 1938), vol. 1: *1889-1919*, 446-47, 464.

88. Dos Passos, *The Fourteenth Chronicle: Letters and Diaries of John Dos Passos*, ed. Townsend Ludington (Boston: Gambit, 1973), 246.

89. Letter dated 8 April 1919, Seymour Papers.

90. Diaries, 4 April 1919, McCormick Papers.

91. Letter dated 13 April 1919, Seymour Papers.

92. U.S. Department of Health, Education, and Welfare, Public Health Service, *Mortality From Influenza and Pneumonia in 50 Large Cities of the United States 1919-1929*, by Selwyn D. Collins, W. H. Frost, Mary Gover, and Edgar Sydenstricker, Reprint no. 1415 from *Public Health Reports* 45, 26 September 1930, p. 32 (Washington, D.C. Government Printing Office, 1930), p. 11.

93. Ibid., 28, 30-31.

94. New York Times, 16, 18 March 1919.

95. Ibid., 30 April 1919.

96. M.A. DeWolfe Howe, *John Jay Chapman and His Letters* (Boston: Houghton Mifflin, 1937): 334.

97. Thomas Wolfe, *Look Homeward, Angel* (New York: Charles Scribner's Sons, 1929, Bantam Edition, 1970): 520.

CHAPTER 6: THE AFTERMATH (1919)

1. Alexander Trachtenberg, ed., *American Labor Yearbook, 1917-18.* (New York: Rand School of Social Science, 1918): 164.

2. New York Times, 18 May 1919.

3. Ibid.

4. Ibid.

5. William H. Peters, *After Effects of Influenza in Cincinnati* (Cincinnati: American Red Cross Health Crusade, 1919): 5-13.

6. Ibid.

7. U.S. Department of Health, Education, and Welfare, Public Health

Service, *Mortality From Influenza and Pneumonia in 50 Large Cities of the United States 1919-1929*, by Selwyn D. Collins, W. H. Frost, Mary Gover, and Edgar Sydenstricker, Reprint no. 1415 from *Public Health Reports* 45, 26 September 1930, p. 32 (Washington, D.C. Government Printing Office, 1930), p. 30.

8. Peters, ibid.

9. Ibid.

10. Ibid.

11. Ibid.

12. Ibid.

13. Ibid.

14. Ibid.

15. Ibid.

16. Ibid.

17. Ibid.

18. Ibid.

19. Ibid.

20. Ibid.

21. Lavinia L. Dock, et al, *History of American Red Cross Nursing* (New York: Macmillan Co., 1922): 979.

22. "Preparedness," Inter-Office Letter dated 11 December 1919, Mountain Division, Denver, Colorado, 1918 Influenza File, #803.031, Library of the American National Red Cross, Washington, D.C.

23. "Social Problems Arising as a Result of Influenza Epidemic," Inter-Office Letter, 25 October 1918, 1918 Influenza File, #803.6, American Red Cross.

24. "Home Services for Victims of Influenza," Letter to Division Managers, 1 March 1919, 1918 Influenza File, #803.6, American Red Cross.

25. Ibid.

26. *New York Times*, 16 December 1918.

27. Dock, 1023-27.

28. "25th Anniversary – Yale School of Nursing," *Yale Journal of Biology and Medicine* (1949): 264-71.

29. Mary Laird, R.N.. to C.-E. A. W., September 4, 1919, C.-E. A. Winslow Papers, Manuscripts and Archives, Yale University Library, New Haven.

30. Ibid.

31. *New York Times*, 19 October 1918.

32. Ibid., 21 October 1918.

33. Ibid., 2 March 1919.

34. Ibid., 8 June 1919.

35. *President's Report 1919-1920* (New Haven: Yale UP, 1920), *Reports of the Presidents of Yale University*, p. 403-10.

36. *New York Times*, 1 June 1919.

37. Ibid.

38. *President's Report 1919-1920* (New Haven: Yale UP, 1920), *Reports of the Presidents of Yale University*, p. 15.

39. *New York Times*, 3 June 1919.

40. Ibid., 6 April 1919.

41. "Appropriation by Congress for Investigation and Combating Influenza" *Journal of the American Medical Association* 73 (1919): 349.

42. Dr. Otto P. Geier to Dr. Harold L. Amoss, letter and enclosures, 29 July 1919, Papers of Harold Lindsay Amoss, Library of the American Philosophical Society, Philadelphia.

43. Ibid.

44. *New York Times*, 18 June 1919.

45. Ibid., 25 September 1918.

46. Ibid.

47. Ibid.

48. "First Meeting of Commission on Influenza Appointed by Gov. Whitman," 30 October 1918, pp. 1-7,

Winslow Papers.

49. Ibid.

50. Ibid.

51. Ibid., 2.

52. Ibid., 2-3.

53. Ibid., 3-4.

54. Ibid.

55. Ibid.

56. Ibid., 5-6.

57. Ibid., 1-7.

58. "Third Meeting of Commission on Influenza Appointed by Gov. Whitman," 20 December 1918, p. 5, Winslow Papers.

59. "Fourth Meeting of Commission on Influenza Appointed by Gov. Whitman," 14 February 1919, p. 3, Winslow Papers.

60. *New York Times*, 13 January 13, 1919.

61. 31 December 1918, Blake Papers.

62. Ibid., 2 January 1919.

63. "Joint Influenza Committee," *Public Health Reports* 34, 28 February 1919, p. 377.

64. American Public Health Association, Section on Vital Statistics, Committee on Statistical Study of the Influenza Epidemic, to C.-E. A. Winslow, 23 November 1918, Winslow Papers.

65. Kenneth F. Maxcy, M.D., *Papers of Wade Hampton Frost, M.D.: A Contribution to Epidemiological Method* (New York: Commonwealth Fund, 1941): 10-13.

66. *New York Times*, 29 September 1918.

67. Ibid., 2 October 1918.

68. Ibid., 31 March 1919.

69. Ibid., 25 December 1918.

70. Ibid., 14 June 1919.

71. Ibid., 3 July, 10, 12 August 1919.

72. Ibid., 15 August 1919.

73. Ibid., 15 August 1919.

74. Ibid., 24 August 1919.

75. Ibid., 14 September 1919.

76. Ibid.

77. Ibid., 21 September 1919.

78. Ibid.

79. Ibid., 29 September 1919.

80. Ibid., 27 September 1919, 3 October 1919.

81. Ibid., 12, 14 October 1919.

82. Ibid., 30 October 1919.

83. Ibid., 15 November 1919.

84. Ibid., 30 November 1919.

CHAPTER 7: A TIRED NATION (1920)

1. *New York Times*, 31 January 1920.

2. Ibid., 1 January 1920.

3. *Washington Post*, 22, 28 December 1919; 9, 19 January 1920.

4. Ibid., 5 January 1920.

5. *New York Times*, 10 January 1920.

6. Ibid., 13 January 1920.

7. 1920 Diary, Diaries 1902-1940, Papers of Raymond Pearl, Library of the American Philosophical Society, Philadelphia.

8. Ibid.

9. Ibid.

10. Robert Frost and Elinor Frost, *Family Letters of Robert and Elinor Frost*, ed. Arnold E. Grade. Albany: State University of New York Press, 1972): 73-75. [Hereafter referred to as Grade.]

11. *Washington Post*, 16 January 1920.

12. Ibid., 15, 20, 23 January 1920.

13. Ibid., 26, 27 January 1920.

14. *New York Times*, 23 January 1920.

15. Letter to Surgeon General, Public Health Service, dated 30 January 1920, from A. W. Hollis, M.D., and C. T. Chetwood, M.D., General Files 1897-

1923, #1622, Records of the Public Health Service, Record Group 90, *National Archives*.

16. *Washington Post*, 28 January 1920.

17. Franklin K. Lane, *The Letters of Franklin K. Lane: Personal and Political*. Edited by Anne Wintermute Lane and Louise Herrick Wall. (Boston: Houghton Mifflin, 1922): 393-94.

18. Belle Case LaFollette and Fola LaFollette, *Robert M. LaFollette*, 2 vols. (New York: Macmillan, 1953): 991-96.

19. Ibid., 854-920.

20. *Washington Post*, 29 January 1920; *Public Health Reports* 35, 12 March 1920, p. 582.

21. *Washington Post*, 29 January 1920.

22. Ibid., 2 March 1920.

23. Ibid., 8, 18 February 1920.

24. Ibid., 21 January 1920.

25. Ibid., 31 January 1920.

26. *Public Health Reports* 35, 12 March 1920, p. 582; *Washington Post*, 29 January 1920; U.S. Department of Health, Education, and Welfare, Public Health Service, *Mortality From Influenza and Pneumonia in 50 Large Cities of the United States 1919-1929*, by Selwyn D. Collins, W. H. Frost, Mary Gover, and Edgar Sydenstricker, Reprint no. 1415 from *Public Health Reports* 45, 26 September 1930, p. 32 (Washington, D.C. Government Printing Office, 1930), p. 13.

27. *New York Times*, 27 January 1920.

28. Ibid., 24 January 1920; *Washington Post* 29 January 1920.

29. *New York Times*, 30 January 1920.

30. *Washington Post*, 29 January 1920; *New York Times*, 7 March 1920.

31. *New York Times*, 31 January 1920.

32. Ibid., 1 February 1920.

33. Ibid., 3 July, 8 August 1920.

34. Ibid., 3 February 1920; *Washington Post*, 11 January, 3 February 1920.

35. *New York Times*, 4 February 1920.

36. Hans Zinsser, "The Etiology and Epidemiology of Influenza," *Medicine* 1 (1922): 296.

37. *New York Times*, 1 February 1920.

38. Ibid., 4 February 1920.

39. *Washington Post*, 5 February 1920.

40. Ibid., 13 January, 8 February 1920.

41. Ibid., 9 February 1920.

42. Ibid., 23 February 1920.

43. *New York Times*, 11 February 1920.

44. Ibid., 28 February, 9 March 1920.

45. Ibid., 2 March 1920.

46. *Washington Post*, 5 March 1920.

47. 1920 Diary, Pearl Papers.

48. Grade, 75-77.

49. Ibid.

50. Robert Frost, *Selected Letters of Robert Frost*. Edited by Lawrence Thompson (New York: Holt, Rinehart and Winston, 1964): 238-41; Robert Frost, *The Letters of Robert Frost to Louis Untermeyer*. Edited by Louis Untermeyer (New York: Holt, Rinehart and Winston, 1963): 114.

51. Ibid.

52. Grade, 96.

53. *New York Times*, 7 March 1920.

54. Ibid., 26 March 1920.

55. Ibid., 2 April 1920.

56. Ibid., 3 April 1920.

57. Ibid., 11 April 1920.

58. Ibid., 14 April 1920; Hughes, Charles Evans, *The Autobiographical Notes of Charles Evans Hughes*. Edited by David J. Danielski and Joseph S. Tulchin (Cambridge: Harvard UP, 1973): 196-97.

59. *New York Times*, 24 May 1920.

60. Ibid., 30 May, 6 June 1920.

61. Ibid., 11 June 1920.

62. Ibid., 19 June 1920; Edward Robb Ellis, *Echoes of Distant Thunder: Life in the United States, 1914-1918* (New York: Coward, McCann & Geoghegan, 1975): 471.

63. *New York Times*, 3 October 1920.

64. Ibid., 4 August 10 November 1920; 3 January 1921.

65. Ibid., 3 November 1920.

66. Frederick Lewis Allen, *Only Yesterday* (New York: Harper & Bros., Bantam Books, 1959): 30.

67. *New York Times*, 3 December 1920.

68. Ibid., 20 December 1920; *Washington Post*, 24 December 1920.

69. *New York Times*, 14 December 1920.

70. Lane and Wall, 377.

71. *New York Times*, 7, 14, 17, 18 December 1920; *Washington Post* 26 December 1920.

72. William Allen White, *Selected Letters of William Allen White 1899-1943*. Edited by Walter Johnson (New York: Henry Holt, 1947): 213.

73. Frederick Lewis Allen, *The Big Change: America Transforms Itself 1900-1950* (New York: Harper, 1952, Bantam, 1961): 118.

74. John Dewey, *Characters and Events: Popular Essays in Social and Political Philosophy*, ed. Joseph Ratner, 2 vols. (New York: Henry Holt, 1929), 2: 760-61.

CHAPTER 8: THE BATTLE CONTINUES

1. Jamie Shreeve, "Why Revive a Deadly Flu Virus?" *New York Times*, 29 January 2006, [n.p.].

2. John M. Barry, "The Site of Origin of the 1918 Influenza Pandemic and its Public Health Implications." *Journal of Translational Medicine* 2, no. 1, 20 January 2004, p. 3.

3. John S. Oxford, "The So-called Great Spanish Influenza Pandemic of 1918 May Have Originated in France in 1916," *Philosophical Transactions of the Royal Society of London. Series B, Biological Sciences* 356, no. 1416, 29 December 2001, pp. 1857-59.

4. John S. Oxford, Robert Lambkin, Armine Sefton, Rod Daniels, Aileen Elliot, R. Brown and D. Gill, "A Hypothesis: The Conjunction of Soldiers, Gas, Pigs, Ducks, Geese and Horses in Northern France During the Great War Provided the Conditions for the Emergence of the 'Spanish' Influenza Pandemic of 1918-1919," *Vaccine* 23, no. 7, 4 January 2005, pp. 940-45.

5. John M. Barry, *Journal of Translational Medicine*; Alfred W. Crosby, *America's Forgotten Pandemic: The Influenza of 1918*. 2nd ed. Cambridge: Cambridge University Press.

6. Jeffrey K. Taubenberger, Ann H. Reid and Thomas G. Fanning, "Capturing a Killer Flu Virus," *Scientific American* 292, no. 1 (January 2005): 62-71

7. Mark J. Gibbs and Adrian J. Gibbs, "Molecular Virology: Was the 1918 Pandemic Caused by a Bird Flu?" *Nature* 440, 27 April 2006, p. E8; Janis Antonovics, Michael E. Hood, Christi H. Baker, "Molecular Virology: Was the 1918 Flu Avian in Origin?" *Nature* 440, no. 7088 (2006): E9.

8. Taubenberger, Reid and Fanning (2005).

9. Terrence M. Tumpey, Christopher F. Basler, Patricia V. Aguilar, Hui Zeng, Alicia Solórzano, David E. Swayne, Nancy J. Cox, Jacqueline M. Katz, Jeffrey

K. Taubenberger, Peter Palese and Adolfo García-Sastro, "Characterization of the Reconstructed 1918 Spanish Influenza Pandemic Virus" *Science* 310, no. 5745, 7 October 2005, pp. 77-80.

10. Eugenia Tognotti, "Scientific Triumphalism and Learning from Facts: Bacteriology and the "Spanish flu" Challenge of 1918," *Social History of Medicine* 16, no. 1 (2003): 97-110.

11. Joshua Lederberg, "H1N1-Influenza as Lazarus: Genomic Resurrection from the Tomb of an Unknown," *Proceedings of the National Academy of Sciences of the United States of America* 98, no. 5, 27 February 2001, pp. 2115-16.

12. Robert B. Belshe, "The Origins of Pandemic Influenza – Lessons from the 1918 Virus," *New England Journal of Medicine* 353, no. 21, 24 November 2005, pp. 2209-11; Iain Stephenson and Jane Democratis, "Influenza: Current Threat From Avian Influenza," *British Medical Bulletin* 75-76, no. 1 (2006): 63-80.

13. Writing Committee of the World Health Organization (WHO) Consultation on Human Influenza A/H5, "Avian Influenza A (H5N1) Infection in Humans," *New England Journal of Medicine* 353, no. 13, 29 September 2005, pp. 1374-85.

14. http://www.who.int/topics/avian_influenza/en/

15. Chandrakant Lahariya, A.K. Sharma and S.K. Pradhan, "Avian Flu and Possible Human Pandemic," *Indian Pediatrics* 43, no. 4 (April 2006): 317-25.

16. W. Wayt Gibbs and Christine Soares, "Preparing for a Pandemic," *Scientific American* 293, no. 5 (November 2005): 45-54.

17. James Stevens, Ola Blixt, Terrence M. Tumpey, Jeffrey K. Taubenberger, James C. Paulson, Ian A. Wilson, "Structure and Receptor Specificity of the Haemagglutinin from an H5N1 Influenza Virus," *Science* 312, no. 5772, 21 April 2006, pp. 404-10.

18. Writing Committee of the World Health Organization (WHO).

19. Belshe, (2005).

20. Stevens, et al., 21 April 2006.

21. James Stevens, Ola Blixt, Glaser L, Jeffrey K. Taubenberger, Peter Palese, James C. Paulson, Ian A. Wilson, "Glycan Microarray Analysis of the Hemagglutinins from Modern and Pandemic Influenza Viruses Reveals Different Receptor Specificities," *Journal of Molecular Biology* 355 (February 2006): 1143-55.

22. Michael J. Lodes, Dominic Suciu, Mark Elliott, Axel G. Stover, Marty Ross, Marcelo Carabello, Kim Dix, James Crye, Richard J. Webby, Wanda J. Lyon, David L. Danley and Andrew McShea, "Use of Semiconductor-Based Oligonucleotide Microarrays for Influenza A Virus Subtype Identification and Sequencing," *Journal of Clinical Microbiology* 44, no. 4 (April 2006): 1209-18.

23. Gibbs & Soares, (2005).

24. Ibid.

25. Neil M. Ferguson, Derek A.T. Cummings, Simon Cauchemez, Christophe Fraser, Steven Riley, Aronrag Meeyai, Sopon Iamsirithaworn and Donald S. Burke, "Strategies for Containing an Emerging Influenza Pandemic in Southeast Asia," *Nature* 437, no. 7056, 3 August 2005, pp. 209-14.

26. Ira M. Longini, Jr., Azhar Nizam, Shufu Xu, Kumnuan Ungchusak, Wanna Hanshaoworakul, Derek A.T. Cummings, M. Elizabeth Halloran, "Containing Pandemic Influenza at the Source," *Science* 309, no. 5737, 3 August 2005, pp. 1083-87. Epub, 3 August 2005.

27. Gibbs & Soares, (2005).

28. Ben S. Cooper, Richard J. Pitman, W. John Edmunds, Nigel J. Gay, "Delaying the International Spread of Pandemic Influenza," *PLoS Medicine* 3, no. 6 (June 2006): e212. Epub, 2 May 2006, ahead of print.

29. John S. Brownstein, Cecily J. Wolfe and Kenneth D. Mandl, "Empirical Evidence for the Effect of Airline Travel on Inter-Regional Influenza Spread in the United States," *PLosMedicine* 3, no. 10 (November 2006): e503. Epub ahead of print.

30. Neil M. Ferguson, Derek A.T. Cummings, Simon Cauchemez, Christophe Fraser, Steven Riley, Aronrag Meeyai, Sopon Iamsirithaworn and Donald S. Burke, "Strategies for Containing an Emerging Influenza Pandemic in Southeast Asia," *Nature* 437, no. 7056, 3 August 2005, pp. 209-14.

31. Tumpey, et al. (2005); Gibbs & Soares (2005).

32. John Oxford, Shobana Balasingham, Rob Lambkin, "A New Millennium Conundrum: How to Use a Powerful Class of Influenza Anti-Neuraminidase Drugs (NAIs) in the Community," *Journal of Antimicrobial Chemotherapy* 53 (2004): 133-36.

33. Menno D. de Jong, Tran Tan Thanh, Truong Huu Khanh, Vo Minh Hien, Gavin J.D. Smith, Nguyen Vinh Chau, Bach Van Cam, et al., "Oseltamivir Resistance During Treatment of Influenza A (H5N1) Infection," *New England Journal of Medicine* 353, no. 25, 22 December 2005, pp. 2667-72.

34. Oxford, et al. (2004).

35. Roland R. Regoes and Sebastian Bonhoeffer, "Emergence of Drug-Resistant Influenza Virus: Population Dynamical Considerations," *Science* 312, no. 5772, 21 April 2006, pp. 389-91.

36. Vasily P. Mishin, Frederick G. Hayden, Larisa V. Gubareva, "Susceptibilities of Antiviral-Resistant Influenza Viruses to Novel Neuraminidase Inhibitors," *Antimicrobial Agents and Chemotherapy* 49, no. 11 (November 2005): 4515-20.

37. Michael P. Malakhov, Laura M. Aschenbrenner, Donald F. Smee, Miles K. Wandersee, Robert W. Sidwell, Larisa V. Gubareva, Vasily P. Mishin, Frederick G. Hayden, Do Hyong Kim, Alice Ing, Erin R. Campbell, Mang Yu and Fang Fang, "Sialidase Fusion Protein as a Novel Broad-Spectrum Inhibitor of Influenza Virus Infection," *Antimicrobial Agents and Chemotherapy* 50, no. 4 (April 2006): 1470-79.

38. Maretta C. Mann, Tasneem Islam, Jeffrey Dyason, Pas Florio, Carolyn J. Trower,Robin J. Thomson, Mark Itstein, "Unsaturated N-Acetyl-D-Glucosaminuronic Acid Glycosides as Inhibitors of Influenza Virus Sialidase," *Glycoconjugate Journal* 23, nos. 1-2 (February 2006): 127-33.

39. Stephen W. Schwarzmann, J.L. Adler, R.J. Sullivan, Jr., William M. Marine, "Bacterial Pneumonia During the Hong Kong Influenza Epidemic of

1968-1969," *Archives of Internal Medicine* 127, no. 6 (June 1971): 1037-41.

40. Marc J.M Bonten and Jan M. Prins, "Antibiotics in Pandemic Flu will be Essential for Treating, but not Preventing, Bacterial Pneumonia," *British Medical Journal* 332, no. 7536, 4 February 2006, pp. 248-49.

41. Fitzhugh Mullan, *Plagues and Politics: The Story of the United States Public Health Service.* New York: Basic Books, 1989. 182-85.

42. Ferguson, et al. (2006).

43. John J. Treanor, James D. Campbell, Kenneth M. Zangwill, Thomas Rowe, M.S. Wolff and Mark Wolff, "Safety and Immunogenicity of an Inactivated Subvirion Influenza A (H5N1) Vaccine," *New England Journal of Medicine* 354, no. 13, 30 March 2006, pp. 1347-51.

44. Gibbs & Soares (2005).

45.Ibid.

46. J.M. Audsley and Gregory A. Tannock, "The Role of Cell Culture Vaccines in the Control of the Next Influenza Pandemic," *Expert Opinion on Biological Therapy* 4, no. 5, 1 May 2004, pp. 709-17; Suzanne L. Epstein, Terrence M. Tumpey, Julia A. Misplon, Chia-Yun Lo, Lynn A. Cooper, Kanta Subbarao, Mary Renshaw, Suryaprakash Sambhara and Jacqueline M. Katz, "DNA Vaccine Expressing Conserved Influenza Virus Proteins Protective Against H5N1 Challenge Infection in Mice," *Emerging Infectious Diseases* 8, no. 8 (August 2002): 796-801.

47. "Regional Update: Prospects for a Pandemic (Winter 2007)." Woodrow Wilson School of Public and International Affairs, Princeton University. http://72.14.209.104/search?q=cache:80fitwpraesJ:region.princeton.edu/issue_120.html+nursing+shortage+influenza+pandemic&hl=en&ct=clnk&cd=9&gl=us

48. Robert G. Webster, "Predictions for Future Human Influenza Pandemics." *Journal of Infectious Diseases* 176, Suppl. 1 (August 1997): S14-19.

49. James E. Hollenbeck, "An Avian Connection as a Catalyst to the 1918-1919 Influenza Pandemic," *International Journal of Medical Sciences* 2, no. 2 (2005): 87-90.

50. "Bird Flu Research Must Be Shared Faster," *New Scientist* 191, no. 2567, 2 September 2006, p. 5.

51. Jeffrey K. Taubenberger and David M. Morens, "1918 Influenza: The Mother of All Pandemic," *Emerging Infectious Diseases* 12.1 (January 2006): 20.

52. Ibid, p.21

Select Bibliography

Because the potential sources of research material relating to the 1918-20 influenza pandemic are seemingly endless, any bibliography would necessarily have to be selective. In the pages that follow, only those sources that were deemed to be pertinent to this study by the authors are listed. The greater part of this study has been drawn from primary sources, in particular manuscript and archive collections, diaries, letters, and memoirs. Of great value, as well, was the periodical medical literature. No history of any period would be complete, of course, without reference to daily newspapers, which often provide the details that make history come alive. Undoubtedly, a wide variety of other interesting resources might have been used to write a history of the pandemic as well.

MANUSCRIPT COLLECTIONS

Oral History Research Office, 801 Butler Library, Columbia University, New York, New York.
 Reminiscences of Dana W. Atchley
 Reminiscences of Dr. Joseph Aub
 Reminiscences of A.R. Dochez
 Reminiscences of Eddie Dowling
 Reminiscences of Miss Caroline King Duer
 Reminiscences of Dr. Alan Gregg
 Reminiscences of Isabel Maitland Stewart
American Philosophical Society Library, Philadelphia, Pennsylvania.
 Harold Lindsay Amoss Papers
 Rufus Ivory Cole Papers
 Simon Flexner Papers
 Victor George Heiser Papers
 Peter K. Olitsky Papers
 Eugene Lindsay Opie Papers
 Raymond Pearl Papers
 Peyton Rous Papers
American Red Cross—National Headquarters Library, Washington, D.C.
 Epidemics, Influenza
Manuscript Division, Library of Congress, Washington, D.C.
 Newton D. Baker Papers
 Ray Stannard Baker Papers
 Bainbridge Colby Papers
 George Creel Papers
 Charles Evans Hughes Papers
 William G. McAdoo Papers
 Joseph P. Tumulty Papers
 Woodrow Wilson Papers
National Archives and Records Service, College Park, Maryland and Washington, D.C.
 Record Group 15: Records of the Veterans Administration
 Record Group 29: Records of the Bureau of the Census
 Record Group 40: General Records of the Department of Commerce
 Record Group 52: Records of the Bureau of Medicine and Surgery
 Record Group 61: Records of the War Industries Board
 Record Group 62: Records of the Council of National Defense
 Record Group 90: Records of the Public Health Service
 Record Group 102: Records of the Children's Bureau

Record Group 112: Records of the Office of the Surgeon General (Army)

Record Group 165: Records of the War Department General and Special Staffs

Record Group 189: Records of the National Academy of Science

Record Group 190: Records of the Bureau of War Risk Litigation Archives and Modern Manuscripts Program, History of Medicine Division, National Library of Medicine, Bethesda, Maryland.

Autobiographical Memoir (Oral History) of Stanhope   Bayne-Jones

Autobiographical Memoir (Oral History) of Shields Warren Private Collection: Dr. John B. Blake, Bethesda, Maryland.

Francis Gilman Blake Papers

Rockefeller University Archives, Rockefeller Archive Center, Sleepy Hollow, New York.

Peter K. Olitsky Papers

Reports of the Director of the Laboratories and the Director of the Hospital, The Rockefeller Institute for Medical Research Manuscripts and Archives, Yale University Library, New Haven, Connecticut

Gordon Auchincloss Papers

Francis Gilman Blake Papers

Clive Day Papers

Irving Fisher Papers

Colonel E.M. House Collection

James M. Howard Papers

Kent Family Papers

Arthur Bliss Lane Papers

Vance C. McCormick Papers

Reports of the Presidents of Yale University

Charles Seymour Papers

Henry Lewis Stimson Diaries 1909-1928

Frederic Collin Walcott Correspondence and Manuscripts

Paul M. Warburg Collection

Charles-Edward A. Winslow Papers

Sir William Wiseman Collection

Alan Mason Chesney Medical Archives, Johns Hopkins Medical Institutions, Baltimore, Maryland.

William H. Welch Papers

DIARIES, LETTERS, MEMOIRS AND NARRATIVES

Baker, Ray Stannard. *American Chronicle: The Autobiography of Ray Stannard Baker (David Grayson)*. New York: Charles Scribner's Sons, 1945.

Barker, Lewellys F. *Time and the Physician: The Autobiography of Lewellys Barker*. New York: G.P. Putnam's Sons, 1942.

Benison, Saul. *Tom Rivers: Reflections on a Life in Medicine and Science*. Cambridge, Mass.: MIT Press, 1967.

Berle, Beatrice Bishop, and Jacobs, Travis Beal. *Navigating the Rapids 1918-1971: From the Papers of Adolf A. Berle*. New York: Harcourt-Brace-Jovanovich, 1973.

Binding, Rudolf. *A Fatalist at War*. Translated by Ian F.D. Morrow. Boston: Houghton Mifflin, 1929.

Blumenson, Martin. *The Patton Papers 1885-1940*. Boston: Houghton Mifflin, 1972.

Boylston, Helen Dore. *"Sister": The War Diary of a Nurse*. New York: Ives Washburn, 1927.

Carson, William G.B. *Dear Josephine: he Theatrical Career of Josephine Hull*. Norman: University of Oklahoma Press, 1965.

Corday, Michael. *The Paris Front: An Unpublished Diary 1914-1918*. New York: E.P. Dutton, 1934.

Crosby, Albert W. *America's Forgotten Pandemic: The Influenza of 1918*. 2d ed. Cambridge: Cambridge University Press, 2003).

Cushing, Harvey. *From A Surgeon's Journal 1915-1918*. Boston: Little, Brown, 1936.

Davis, Loyal. *A Surgeon's Odyssey*. Garden City, N.Y.: Doubleday, 1973.

Dos Passos, John. *The Fourteenth Chronicle: Letters and Diaries of John Dos Passos*. Edited by Townsend Ludington. Boston: Gambit, 1973.

Duffy, John. *Epidemics in Colonial America*. Baton Rouge: Louisiana State University Press, 1953.

Frost, Robert. *The Letters of Robert Frost to Louis Untermeyer*. Edited by Louis Untermeyer. New York: Holt, Rinehart & Winston, 1963.

_____. *Selected Letters of Robert Frost*. Edited by Lawrance Thompson. New York: Holt, Rinehart & Winston, 1964.

Frost, Robert and Elinor. *Family Letters of Robert and Elinor Frost*. Compiled and edited by Arnold Grade and with a foreword by Lesley Frost. Albany: State University of New York Press, 1972.

Fulton, John F. *Harvey Cushing: A Biography*. Springfield, Ill.: Charles C. Thomas, 1946.

George, Lloyd. *Memoirs of the Peace Conference*. New Haven: Yale University Press, 1939.

Gleaves, Albert. *A History of the Transport Service: Adventures and Experiences of U.S. Transports and Cruisers in the World War*. New York: George H. Doran, 1921.

Grew, Joseph C. *Turbulent Era: A Diplomatic Record of Forty Years 1904-1945*. Boston: Houghton Mifflin, 1952.

Harriman, Mrs. J. Borden. *From Pinafores to Politics*. New York: Henry Holt, 1923.

Herrick, James B. *Memories of Eighty Years*. Chicago: University of Chicago Press, 1949.

Hodgins, Eric. *Trolley to the Moon: An Autobiography*. New York: Simon & Schuster, 1974.

Hoover, Herbert. *The Memoirs of Herbert Hoover: Years of Adventure 1874-1920*. New York: Macmillan, 1951.

Hoover, Irwin Hood (Ike). *Forty-Two Years in the White House*. Boston: Houghton Mifflin, 1934.

Hopkins, Arthur W., M.D. *Pep, Pills, and Politics: An Odyssey of Two States*. Brattleboro: Vermont Printing, 1944.

House, Edward Mandell. *The Intimate Papers of Colonel House: The Ending of the War*. Arranged as a narrative by Charles Seymour. Boston: Houghton-Mifflin, 1928.

Howe, M.A. DeWolfe. *John Jay Chapman and His Letters*. Boston: Houghton Mifflin, 1937.

Hughes, Charles Evans. *The Autobiographical Notes of Charles Evans Hughes*. Edited by David J. Danielski and Joseph S. Tulchin. Studies in Legal History Series. Cambridge: Harvard University Press, 1973.

Keyes, Frances Parkinson. *All Flags Flying: Reminiscences of Frances Parkinson Keyes*. New York: McGraw-Hill, 1972.

Klein, Daryl. *With the Chinks*. London: John Lane, 1919.

Kuncz, Aladar. *Black Monastery*. Translated by Ralph Murray. New York: Harcourt, Brace, 1934. LaFollette, Belle Case, and Fola Follette. *Robert M. LaFollette*. 2 vols. New York: Macmillan, 1953.

Lane, Franklin K. *The Letters of Franklin K. Lane: Personal and Political*. Edited by Anne Wintermute Lane and Louise Herrick Wall. Boston: Houghton Mifflin, 1922.

Lash, Joseph P. *Eleanor and Franklin: The Story of Their Relationship Based on Eleanor Roosevelt's Private Papers*. New York: W.W. Norton, 1971. La Gallienne, Eva. *At 33*. New York: Longmans, Green, 1934.

MacCallum, W.G. "Biographical Memoir of Harvey Cushing," in *Biographical Memoirs* of the National Academy of Sciences of the United States of America, Vol. 23. Washington, D.C.: National Academy of Sciences, 1943.

Martin, Dr. Franklin H. *Fifty Years of Medicine and Surgery: An Autobiographical Sketch*. Chicago: Surgical Publishing, 1934.

Morgenthau, Henry. *All in a Life-Time*. With French Strother. Garden City, N.Y.: Doubleday, Page, 922.

Pershing, John J. *My Experiences in the World War*. 2 vols. New York: Frederick A. Stokes, 1931. Richberg, Donald. *My Hero: The Indiscreet Memoirs of an Eventful but Unheroic Life: An Autobiography*. New York: G.P. Putnam's Sons, 1954.

Roosevelt, Franklin D., *F.D.R.: His Personal Letters 1905-1928*. Edited by Elliot Roosevelt, assisted by James N. Rosenau. Foreword by Eleanor Roosevelt. New York: Duell, Sloan & Pearce, 1948.

St. John, Robert. *This Was My World*. Garden City, N.Y.: Doubleday, 1953.

Steed, Henry Wickham. *Through Thirty Years 1892-1922: A Personal Narrative*. 2 vols. Garden City, N.Y.: Doubleday, Page, 1924.

Steffens, Lincoln. *The Letters of Lincoln Steffens*. 2 vols. Edited by Ella Winter and Granville Hicks, with a memorandum by Carl

Sandburg. New York: Harcourt, Brace, 1938.

Stevenson, Adlai. *The Papers of Adlai*
E. Stevenson. Edited by Walter Johnson. 2 vols. Boston: Little, Brown, 1972.

Vaughn, Victor C. *A Doctor's Memories.* Indianapolis: Bobbs-Merrill, 1926.

White, William Allen. *Selected Letters of William Allen White 1899- 1943.* Edited by
Walter Johnson. New York: Henry Holt, 1947.

Wu Lien-teh. *Plague Fighter: The Autobiography of a Modern Chinese Physician.*
Cambridge, England: W. Heffer and Sons, 1959.

Young, Hugh. *Hugh Young: A Surgeon's Autobiography.* New York: Harcourt, Brace,
1940.

Zinsser, Hans. *As I Remember Him: The Biography of R.S.* Boston: Little, Brown, 1940.

SPECIAL STUDIES, MONOGRAPHS, AND GENERAL LITERATURE

Ackerknecht, Erwin H., *History and Geography of the Most Important Diseases.* New
York: Hafner, 1965.

Adams, John M., *Viruses and Colds: The Modern Plague.* New York: American Elsevier,
1967.

Allen, Frederick Lewis. *Only Yesterday.* New York: Harper Bros., 1931.

_____. *The Big Change: America Transforms Itself 1900-1950.* New York: Harper,
1952.

Alpert, Hollis. *The Barrymores.* New York: Dial Press, 1964.

Ashburn, P.M., *A History of the Medical Department of the United States Army.* Boston:
Houghton Mifflin, 1929.

Baker, Ray Stannard. *Woodrow Wilson: Life and Letters.* New York: Doubleday, Doran
& Co., 1939.

Barry, John M., *The Great Influenza: The Epic Story of the Deadliest Plague in History.*
New York: Viking Penguin, 2004.

Barry, John M., 1918 Revisited: Lessons and Suggestions for Further Inquiry in
"The Threat of Pandemic Influenza Are we Ready?" Workshop Summary. Ed. S.L.
Knobler. Washington D.C.: National Academies Press, 2005. 66.

Beaver, Daniel R. *Newton D. Baker and the American War Effort 1917-19.* Lincoln:
University of Nebraska Press, 1966.

Beaveridge, W.I.B., *Influenza: The Last Great Plague, An Unfinished Story of Discovery.*
New York: Prodist, 1977.

Blanton, Wyndham B., M.D. *Medicine in Virginia in the Seventeenth Century.* Richmond:
William Byrd Press, 1930.

Blick, Judith. "The Chinese Labor Corps in World War I." *Papers on China.*
East Asia Regional Studies Seminar Series, No. 9. Cambridge: Harvard University
Press, 1955.

Buley, R. Carlyle. *The American Life Convention 1906-1952: A Study in the History of
Life Insurance.* 2 vols. New York: Appleton-Century-Crofts, 1953.

Burnet, F.M. and Ellen Clark, *Influenza: A Survey of the Last 50 Years in the Light of Modern Work on the Virus of Epidemic Influenza*. Monographs of the Walter and Eliza Hall Institute of Research in Pathology and Medicine, Melbourne, No. 4. Melbourne: Macmillan, 1942.

Cadbury, William Warden, M.D. *The 1918 Pandemic of Influenza in Canton, China*. Bulletin No. 22. Canton: Canton Christian College, 1919.

Coffman, Edward M. *The War to End all Wars: The American Militarry Experience in World War I*. New York: Oxford University Press, 1968.

Collier, Richard. *The Plague of the Spanish Lady: The Influenza Pandemic of 1918-1919*. New York: Atheneum, 1974. Corner, George W. *A History of the Rockefeller Institute*. New York: Rockefeller Institute Press, 1964.

Crowell, Benedict, and Wilson, Robert Forrest. *How America Went to War. The Road to France*. Vol. 2. New Haven: Yale University Press, 1921.

Dewey, John. *Characters and Events: Popular Essays in Social and Political Philosophy*. 2 vols. Edited by Joseph Ratner. New York: Henry Holt, 1929.

Dock, Lavinia L., Sarah Elizabeth Pickett, Clara D. Noyes, Fannie F. Clement. Elizabeth G. Fox, and Anna R. Van Meter. *History of American Red Cross Nursing*. New York: Macmillan, 1922.

Dos Passos, John. *Mr. Wilson's War*. Mainstream of America Series. Edited by Lewis Gannett. Garden City, N.Y.: Doubleday, 1962.

_____. *Nineteen Nineteen*. Boston: Houghton Mifflin, 1932, Signet Classic, New American Library Edition, 1969. Dublin, Louis I. and Alfred J. Lotka, *Twenty-Five Years of Health Progress: A Study of the Mortality Experience Among the Industrial Policyholders of the Metropolitan Life Insurance Company 1911 to 1935*. New York: Metropolitan Life Insurance, 1937.

Dublin, Louis I. *A Family of Thirty Million: The Story of the Metropolitan Life Insurance Company*. New York: Metropolitan Life Insurance, 1943.

Duffy, John. *Epidemics in Colonial America*. Baton Rouge: Louisiana State University Press, 1953.

Easterday, Robert C., "Influenza," in *Diseases Transmitted From Animals to Man*. Edited by William T. Hubbert, William F. McCulloch, Paul R. Schnurrenberger and Thomas G. Hull. 6th ed. Springfield, Ill.: Charles C. Thomas, 1975.

Ellis, Edward Robb. *Echoes of Distant Thunder: Life in the United States, 1914-1918*. New York: Coward, McCann & Geoghegan, 1975.

Ewald, Paul. *The Evolution of Infectious Disease*. New York: Oxford University Press, 1994.

Ewing, Cortez A.M. *Congressional Elections 1896-1944: The Sectional Basis of Political Democracy in the House of Representatives*. Norman: University of Oklahoma Press, 1947.

Falls, Cyril. *The Great War 1914-18*. New York: G.P. Putnam's Sons, 1959.

Fleming, Donald. *William H. Welch and the Rise of Modern Medicine*. Library of American Biography Series. Edited by Oscar Handlin. Boston: Little, Brown, 1954.

Flexner, Simon, and James Thomas Flexner. *William Henry Welch and the Heroic Age of American Medicine.* New York: Viking Press, 1941.

Gallagher, Richard *Diseases That Plague Modern Man: A History of The Communicable Diseases.* Dobbs Ferry, N.Y.: Oceana Publications, 1969.

Garraty, John A. *Woodrow Wilson: A Great Life in Brief.* Great Lives in Brief Series. New York: Alfred A. Knopf, 1956.

Garrett, Laurie. *The Coming Plague: Newly Emerging Diseases in a World Out of Balance.* New York: Farrar, Straus and Giroux, 1994.

Gelfand, Lawrence E. *The Inquiry: American Preparations for Peace 1917-1919.* New Haven, Conn.: Yale University Press, 1963.

Grayson, Cary T. *Woodrow Wilson: An Intimate Memoir.* New York: Holt, Rinehart & Winston, 1960.

Hagan, William Arthur, and Dorsey William Bruner. *Infectious Diseases of Domestic Animals: With Special Reference to Etiology, Diagnosis, and Biologic Therapy.* 3rd ed. Ithaca, NY: Comstock, 1957.

Hare, Ronald. *Pomp and Pestilence: Infectious Disease, Its Origins and Conquest.* New York: Philosophical Library, 1955.

Hill, Justina Hamilton. *Silent Enemies: The Story of the Diseases of War and Their Control.* New York: Commonwealth Fund, 1941.

Hoehling, A.A. *The Great Epidemic.* Boston: Little, Brown, 1961.

Hoover, Herbert. *America's First Crusade.* New York: Charles Scribner's Sons, 1942.

————. *The Ordeal of Woodrow Wilson.* New York: McGraw-Hill, 1958.

Hoyle, Leslie. *The Influenza Viruses.* Virology Monograph No. 4. *Continuing Handbook of Virology Research.* Edited by S. Gard, C. Hallauer, and K.F. Myer. New York: Springer-Verlag, 1968.

Hubbert, W.T., William F. McCulloch, and Paul R. Schnurrenberger, *Diseases Transmitted from Animals to Man.* Springfield, Ill.: Charles C. Thomas, 1930. 6th ed. 1975.

James, Marquis. *The Metropolitan Life: A Study in Business Growth.* New York: Viking Press, 1947.

Jordan, Edwin O. *Epidemic Influenza: A Survey.* Chicago: American Medical Association, 1927.

Kilbourne, Edwin D., "A Virologist's Perspective on the 1918-1919 Pandemic," in *The Spanish Influenza Pandemic of 1918-19: New Perspectives,* ed. Howard Phillips and David Killingray. New York: Routledge, 2003.

Knight, Vernon and Julius A. Kasel, "Influenza Viruses," in *Viral and Mycoplasmal Infections of the Respiratory Tract.* Edited by Vernon Knight. Philadelphia: Lea & Febinger, 1973.

Gina Kolata. *Flu: The Story of the Great Influenza Pandemic of 1918 and the Search for the Virus that Caused It.* New York: Touchstone Press, 2001.

Livermore, Seward W. *Politics Is Adjourned: Woodrow Wilson and the War Congress 1916-1918.* Middleton, Conn.: Wesleyan University Press, 1966.

Loosli, Clayton G., Bernard Portnoy, and Edna C. Myers. *International Bibliography of Influenza, 1930-1959.*
Los Angeles University of Southern California, School of Medicine, 1978.

MacNair, Harvey Farnsworth. *The Chinese Abroad, Their Position and Protection: A Study in International Law and Relations.* Shanghai: Commercial Press, 1924.

Maxcy, Kenneth F., M.D. *Papers of Wade Hampton Frost, M.D.: A Contribution to Epidemiological Method.* New York: Commonwealth Fund, 1941.

May, Earl Chapin, and Will Oursler. *The Prudential: A Story of Human Security.* Garden City, N.Y.: Doubleday, 1950.

Mencken, H.L. *Minority Report: H.L. Mencken's Notebooks.* New York: Alfred A. Knopf, 1956.

The Mobilization of the American National Red Cross during the Influenza Pandemic 1918–1919. Geneva, Switzerland, 1920.

Mowatt, Charles Loch. *Britain Between the Wars 1918-1940.* Chicago: University of Chicago Press, 1955.

Mulder, Jacob, and J.F. Hers. *Influenza.* Foreword by Sir Charles H. Stewart- Harris. Groningen: Neth.: Wolters-Noordhoff Publishing, 1972.

Mullan, Fitzhugh, *Plagues and Politics: The Story of the United States Public Health Service.* New York: Basic Books, 1989. 182-85.

Muller, Jurgen. "Bibliography," in *TheSpanish Influenza Pandemic of 1918-19: New Perspectives,* ed. Howard Phillips and David Killingray. New York: Routledge, 2003. 301-51.

Opie, Eugene L., Frances G. Blake, James C. Small, and Thomas M. Rivers. *Epidemic Respiratory Disease: The Pneumonias and Other Infections of the Respiratory Tract Accompanying Influenza and Measles.* St. Louis: C.V. Mosby, 1921.

Palmer, Frederick. *Newton D. Baker: America at War.* 2 vols. New York: Dodd, Mead, 1931.

Peters, William H., *After Effects of Influenza in Cincinnati.* Cincinnati: American Red Cross Health Crusade, 1919.

Phillips, Howard and David Killingray, eds. *The Spanish Influenza Pandemic of 1918-19: New Perspectives.* New York: Routledge, 2003.

Pitt, Barrie. *1918: The Last Act.* New York: W.W. Norton, 1962.

Porter, Katherine Anne. "Pale Horse Pale Rider." *Collected Stories of Katherine Anne Porter.* New York: Harcourt, Brace & World, New American Library, 1970.

Rivers, Thomas M., Wendell M. Stanley, Louis O. Kunkel, Richard E. Shope, and Frank L. Horsfall, Jr. *Virus Diseases.* Ithaca, N.Y.: Cornell University Press, 1943.

Seymour, Charles. *Woodrow Wilson and the World War: A Chronicle of Our Own Times.* The Chronicles of America Series, No. 48. Edited by Allen Johnson. New Haven: Yale University Press, 1921.

Shryock, Richard Harrison. *The Development of Modern Medicine: An Interpretation of the Social and Scientific Factors Involved.* London: Victor Gollancz, 1948.

Simonsen, Lone, Thomas A. Reichert, and Mark A. Miller. In *Options for the Control of Influenza V*, ed. Yoshihiro Kawaoka. International Congress Series, no. 1263 (Okinawa Japan: Elsevier, 2003): 791-794.

Sisley, Richard, *Epidemic Influenza: Notes on Its Origin and Method of Spread*. London: Longmans, Green, 1891.

Smith, Geddes. *Plague on Us*. New York: Commonwealth Fund, 1941.

Smith, Gene. *When the Cheering Stopped: The Last Years of Woodrow Wilson*. Introduction by Allan Nevins. New York: William Morrow & Co., 1964.

Stedman's Medical Dictionary for the Health Professions and Nursing. Illus. 5th ed. Philadelphia: Lippincott Williams & Wilkins, 2005.

Stuart-Harris, C.H., *Influenza and Other Viruses: Infections of the Respiratory Tract*. Baltimore: Williams & Wilkins, 1965.

Sullivan, Mark. *Our Times: The United States 1900-1925*. 6 vols. New York: Charles Scribner's Sons, 1933.

Thomson, David, and Thomson, Robert. *Influenza. Pickett-Thomson Research Laboratory Annals*. Vol. 9-10. Baltimore: Williams & Wilkins, 1933.

Trachtenberg, Alexander, ed. *The American Labor Yearbook 1917-18*. New York: Rand School of Social Science, 1918.

Tumulty, Joseph P. *Woodrow Wilson As I Know Him*. Garden City, N.Y.: Doubleday, Page, 1921.

Van Hartesveldt, Fred R. *The 1918-1919 Pandemic of Influenza : The Urban Impact in the Western World*. Lewiston, NY: Edwin Mellen Press, 1992.

Virus and Rickettsial Diseases: With Especial Consideration of Their Public Health Significance. Harvard School of Public Health Symposium, 12-17 June 1939. Cambridge: Harvard University Press, 1940.

Walworth, Arthur. *Woodrow Wilson*. 2 vols. New York: Longmans, Green, 1958.

Williams, Ralph Chester. *The United States Public Health Service 1798-1950*. Washington, D.C.: Commissioned Officers Association of the U.S.P.H.S., 1951.

Wilson, Graham Selby, and A. Ashley Miles, *Topley and Wilson's Principles of Bacteriology and Immunology*, 2 vols. 5th ed. London: Edward Arnold, 1966.

Winslow, C.-E.A. [Charles-Edward Armory]. *The Life of Hermann M. Biggs, M.D., D.Sc., LL.D.: Physician and Statesman of the Public Health*. Philadelphia: Lea & Febiger, 1929.

Winternitz, M.C., Isabel M. Watson, and Frank P. McNamara. *The Pathology of Influenza*. New Haven, Conn.: Yale University Press, 1920.

Thomas Wolfe. *Look Homeward, Angel*. New York: Charles Scribner's Sons, 1929, Bantam Edition, 1970.

PERIODICAL LITERATURE

Articles in the periodical literature which seemed most helpful are found cited below. Medical journals for 1918 and thereafter have a wealth of material on the history of influenza.

Andrewes, Christopher, Patrick P.
  Laidlaw, and Wilson Smith,
  "Influenza: Observations
  on the Recovery of Virus from Man and on the Antibody Content of Human
  Sera." *British Journal of Experimental Pathology* 17 (1935), 579-581.
Antonovics, Janis, Michael E. Hood,
  Christi H. Baker, Molecular Virology:
  Was the 1918 Flu Avian in Origin?" *Nature* 440, no. 7088 (2006): E9.
"Appropriation by Congress for
  Investigation and Combating
  Influenza." *Journal of the American Medical Association* 73 (1919): 349.
Audsley, J.M. and Gregory A.
  Tannock, "The Role of Cell Culture
  Vaccines in the Control of the Next Influenza Pandemic," *Expert Opinion on
  Biological Therapy* 4, no. 5, 1 May 2004, pp. 709-17
Barry, John M. "The Site of Origin of
  the 1918 Influenza Pandemic and its Public Health Implications." *Journal of
  Translational Medicine* 2, no. 1, 20 January 2004, p. 3.
Belshe, Robert B., "The Origins of Pandemic Influenza – Lessons
  from the 1918 Virus," *New England Journal of Medicine* 353, no. 21, 24 November
  2005, pp. 2209-11.
"Bird Flu Research Must Be Shared Faster," *New Scientist* 191, no. 2567, 2
  September 2006, p. 5.
Bonten, Marc J.M., and Jan M. Prins, "Antibiotics in Pandemic Flu will be Essential
  for Treating, but not Preventing, Bacterial Pneumonia," *British Medical Journal* 332,
  no. 7536, 4 February 2006, pp. 248-49.
Brownstein, John S., Cecily J. Wolfe and Kenneth D. Mandl,
  "Empirical Evidence for the Effect of Airline Travel on Inter-Regional Influenza
  Spread in the United States," *PLosMedicine* 3, no. 10 (November 2006): e503.
  Epub ahead of print.
Brundage, John F. "Interactions Between Influenza and Bacterial
  Respiratory Pathogens: Implications for Pandemic Preparedness." *Lancet
  Infectious Diseases* 6, no. 5 (May 2006): 303-12.
Carter, William A. and Erik De Clercq, "Viral Infection and Host
  Defense." *Science* 186 no. 4170, 27 December 1974, 1172-78.
Caulfield, Ernest. "The Pursuit of a Pestilence." *Proceedings of the American*

Antiquarian Society, 1951, 60: 21-52.

Lahariya, Chandrakant, A.K. Sharma and S.K. Pradhan, "Avian Flu
and Possible Human Pandemic," *Indian Pediatrics* 43, no. 4 (April 2006): 317-25.

Chen, Weisan, Paul A. Calvo, Daniela Malide, James Gibbs, Ulrich
Schubert, Igor Bacik, Sameh Basta, et al., "A Novel Influenza A Virus
Mitochondrial Protein that Induces Cell Death." *Nature Medicine* 7 (2001): 1306-12.

"Closing of Moving Picture Shows for Influenza (Alden v. State
Ariz.) 179 *Pac.R.* 646." *Journal of the American Medical Association* 73 (1919): 1007.

Conner, Lewis A., M.D. "The Symptomology and Complications of
Influenza." *Journal of the American Medical Association* 73 (1919): 321-24.

Cooper, Ben S., Richard J. Pitman, W. John Edmunds, Nigel J. Gay,
"Delaying the International Spread of Pandemic Influenza," *PLoS Medicine* 3, no.
6 (June 2006): e212. Epub, 2 May 2006, ahead of print.

De Jong, Menno D., Tran Tan Thanh, Truong Huu Khanh, Vo
Minh Hien, Gavin J.D. Smith, Nguyen Vinh Chau, Bach Van Cam, et al.,
"Oseltamivir Resistance During Treatment of Influenza A (H5N1) Infection,"
New England Journal of Medicine 353, no. 25, 22 December 2005, pp. 2667-72.

Doty, Permelia Murnan. "A Retrospect
of the Influenza Epidemic."
Public Health Nurse 11, no 12 (1919): 949-57.

Douall, James A., and Anne M.
Bahlke, "Epidemic Influenza: A
Comparison of Clinical Observations in a Major and a Minor Epidemic."
American Journal of Hygiene 17 (1933): 562-80. Doucette, Karen E., and Fred Y.
Aoki. "Oseltamivir: A Clinical and Pharmacological Perspective." *Expert Opinion
on Pharmacotherapy* 2, no. 10 (October 2001): 1671-83.

Dowdle, Walter R. "Influenza Pandemic Periodicity, Virus Recycling, and the Art
of Risk Assessment." *Emerging Infectiuous Diseases* 12, no. 1 (January 2006): 34-39.

Easterday, B.C. "Swine Influenza: Historical Perspectives." *Proceedings of the 4th
International Symposium on Emerging and Re-emerging Pig Diseases.* Rome, Italy, 29 June
– 2 July, 2003: pp. 241-44.

Eccles, Ronald. "Understanding the Symptoms of the Common Cold and
Influenza." *Lancet Infectious Diseases* 5, no. 11 (November 2005): 718-725; "The
Epidemic in Shansi: Pneumonic Plague or Influenza?" *China Medical Journal* 33
(1919): 169-73.

Epstein, Suzanne L., Terrence M. Tumpey, Julia A. Misplon, Chia-Yun Lo, Lynn
A. Cooper, Kanta Subbarao, Mary Renshaw, Suryaprakash Sambhara and Jacqueline
M. Katz, "DNA Vaccine Expressing Conserved Influenza Virus Proteins Protective
Against H5N1 Challenge Infection in Mice," *Emerging Infectious Diseases* 8, no. 8
(August 2002): 796-801.

Ferguson, Neil M. Derek A.T. Cummings, Simon Cauchemez, Christophe Fraser,

Steven Riley, Aronrag Meeyai, Sopon Iamsirithaworn and Donald S. Burke, "Strategies for Containing an Emerging Influenza Pandemic in Southeast Asia," *Nature* 437, no. 7056, 3 August 2005, pp. 209-14.

Foley, Edna L., "Department of Public Health Nursing in Charge of Edna L Foley." *American Journal of Nursing* 19, no. 3 (1918): 189-95.

Friedlander, Alfred, Carey P. McCord, Frank J. Sladen, and George W. Wheeler, "The Epidemic of Influenza at Camp Sherman, Ohio." *Journal of the American Medical Association* 71 (1918): 1652-55.

Gamboa, Eugenia T., Abner Wold, Melvin D. Yahr, Donald H. Harter, Phillip E. Duffy, Herbert Barden and Konrad Hsu. "Influenza Virus Antigen in Postencephalitic Parkinsonism Brain." *Archives of Neurology* 51 (October 1974): 228-32.

Garcia-Sastre, Adolfo. "Antiviral Response in Pandemic Influenza Viruses." *Emerging Infectious Diseases* 12, no. 1 (January 2006): 44-47.

Geiss, Gary K., Mirella Salvatore, Terrence M. Tumpey, Victoria S. Carter, Xiuyan Wang, Christopher F. Basler, Jeffrey K. Taubenberger, Roger E. Bumgarner, Peter Palese, Michael G. Katze, Adolofo Garcia-Sastre, "Cellular Transcriptional Profiling in Influenza A Virus-infected Lung Epithelial Cells: The Role of the Nonstructural NS1 Protein in the Evasion of the Host Innate Defense and its Potential Contribution to Pandemic Influenza." *Proceedings of the National Academy of Sciences of the United States of America* 99, no. 16, 6 August 2002, 10736-41.

Gibbs, Mark J. and Adrian J. Gibbs, "Molecular Virology: Was the 1918 Pandemic Caused by a Bird Flu?" *Nature* 440, 27 April 2006, p. E8.

Gibbs, W. Wayt and Christine Soares, "Preparing for a Pandemic," *Scientific American* 293, no. 5 (November 2005): 45-54.

Gibson, H.G., F.B. Bowman, and J.L Connor. *British Medical Journal* (1918) ii, 645.

Gilbreath, Olive. "The Coolie Ship." *Asia* 18 (June 1918): 459-64.

Gill, Charles C. "Overseas Transportation of United States Troops." *Current History* 9: 409-12.

Goodpasture, Ernest W. "The Significance of Certain Pulmonary Lesions in Relation to the Etiology of Influenza." *American Journal of the Medical Sciences* 158 (1919): 863-70.

Gordon, Arthur. "Mental Disorders Following Influenza." *Archives of Internal Medicine* 24 (1919): 633-37.

Greenway, James C., Carl Boettiger and Howard S. Colwell. "Pneumonia and Some of Its Complications at Camp Bowie." *Archives of Internal Medicine* 24 (1919): 1-34.

Gull, B. Manico. "The Story of the Chinese Labor Corps." *Far Eastern Review* 15 (April 1918): 125-35.

Hart, Albert Bushnell. "Baker and His Task." *New York Times*, 7 April 1918,

Magazine Section, pp. 1-2.

Hirshberg, Leonard Keene. "The Spanish Influenza." *Munsey's Magazine* 65 (1918): 64-68.

Hollenbeck, James E. "An Avian Connection as a Catalyst to the 1918-1919 Influenza Pandemic," *International Journal of Medical Sciences* 2, no. 2 (2005): 87-90.

Holmes, Edward C., Jeffrey K. Taubenberger and Bryan T. Grenfell, "Heading Off an Influenza Pandemic," *Science* 309, no. 5737, 12 August, p. 989.

"Investigation and Prevention of Influenza." *Journal of the American Medical Association* 73 (1919): 1146.

"Is the Influenza a Chinese Plague?" *Literary Digest* 59, 7 December 1918, 26-27.

"Joint Influenza Committee." *Public Health Reports* 34, 28 February 1919, p. 377.

Jordan, Edwin O., and W.B. Sharp. "Influenza Studies: Immunity in Influenza." *Journal of Infectious Diseases* 26 (1920): 463-68.

Katz, Robert S. "Influenza 1918-1919: A Study in Mortality." *Bulletin of the History of Medicine* 48 (1974): 416-22.

Kilbourne, Edwin D., "Flu to the Starboard! Man the Harpoons! Fill 'em with Vaccine! Get the Captain! Hurry!" *New York Times*, 13 February 1976.

Kobasa, Darwyn, Ayato Takada, Kyoko Shinya, Masato Hatta, Peter Halfmann, Steven Theriault, Hirishi Suzuki, et al., "Enhanced Virulence of Influenza A Viruses with the Haemagglutinin of the 1918 Pandemic Virus." *Nature* 431, 7 October 2004, 703-707.

_____, Steven M. Jones, Kyoko Shinya, John C. Kash, John Copps, Hideki Ebihara, Yasuko Hatta, Jin Hyun Kim, Peter Halfmann, Masato Hatta, Friederike Feldmann, Judie B. Alimonti, Lisa Fernando, Yan Li, Michael G. Katze, Heinz Feldmann and Yoshihiro Kawaoka, "Aberrant Innate Immune Response in Lethal Injection of Macaques with the 1918 Influenza Virus." *Nature* 445, 18 January 2007, pp. 319-323.

Kotz, A.L. "The Recent Epidemic of Influenza and Brocho-pneumonia at the Easton Hospital, Easton, Pa.: Bacterial Findings A Bacillus Resembling the Bacillus Pestis." *Journal of Laboratory and Clinical Medicine* 4 (April 1919): 424.

Lederberg, Joshua, "H1N1-Influenza as Lazarus: Genomic Resurrection from the Tomb of an Unknown," *Proceedings of the National Academy of Sciences of the United States of America* 98, no. 5, 27 February 2001, pp. 2115-16.

Lee, S.T. "Some of the Different Aspects Between Influenza, Pneumonia, and Pneumonic Plague." *New York Medical Journal* 110, 6 September 1919, 401-03.

Lo, K.C., Jennian F. Geddes, Rod S. Daniels, and John S. Oxford. "Lack of Detection of Influenza Genes in Archived Formalin-fixed, Paraffin Wax-embedded Brain Samples of Encephalitis Lethargica Patients from 1916 to 1920." *Virchows Archiv* 442, no. 6 (June 2003): 591-96.

Lodes, Michael J., Dominic Suciu, Mark Elliott, Axel G. Stover, Marty Ross, Marcelo Carabello, Kim Dix, James Crye, Richard J. Webby, Wanda J. Lyon, David L. Danley and Andrew McShea, "Use of Semiconductor-Based Oligonucleotide Microarrays for Influenza A Virus Subtype Identification and Sequencing," *Journal of Clinical Microbiology* 44, no. 4 (April 2006): 1209-18.

Longini, Ira M., Jr., Azhar Nizam, Shufu Xu, Kumnuan Ungchusak, Wanna Hanshaoworakul, Derek A.T. Cummings, M. Elizabeth Halloran, "Containing Pandemic Influenza at the Source," *Science* 309, no. 5737, 3 August 2005, pp. 1083-87. Epub, 3 August 2005.

Lowy, R. Joel. "Influenza Virus Induction of Apoptosis by Intrinsic and Extrinsic Mechanisms." *International Reviews of Immunology* 22, nos. 5-6, (2003): 425-449.

MacNeal, Ward J. "The Influenza Epidemic of 1918 in the American Expeditionary Forces in France and England." *Archives of Internal Medicine* 23 (1919): 657-88.

McCall, Sherman, James M. Henry, Ann H. Reid, and Jeffrey K. Taubenberger. "Influenza RNA Not Detected in Archival Brain Tissues from Acute Encephalitis Lethargica Cases or in Postencephalitic Parkinson Cases." *Journal of Neuropathology and Experimental Pathology,* 60, no. 7 (July 2001): 696-704.

McCullers, Jonathan A. "Insights into the Interaction Between Influenza Virus and Pneumococcus." *Clinical Microbiology Reviews* 19, no. 3 (July 2006): 571-82.

Malakhov, Michael P., Laura M. Aschenbrenner, Donald F. Smee, Miles K. Wandersee, Robert W. Sidwell, Larisa V. Gubareva, Vasily P. Mishin, Frederick G. Hayden, Do Hyong Kim, Alice Ing, Erin R. Campbell, Mang Yu and Fang Fang, "Sialidase Fusion Protein as a Novel Broad-Spectrum Inhibitor of Influenza Virus Infection," *Antimicrobial Agents and Chemotherapy* 50, no. 4 (April 2006): 1470-79.

Mann, Maretta C., Tasneem Islam, Jeffrey Dyason, Pas Florio, Carolyn J. Trower, Robin J. Thomson, Mark Itstein, "Unsaturated N-Acetyl-D-Glucosaminuronic Acid Glycosides as Inhibitors of Influenza Virus Sialidase," *Glycoconjugate Journal* 23, nos. 1-2 (February 2006): 127-33.

Marine, William M. and Wilton M. Workman. "Hong Kong Influenza Immunologic Recapitulation." *American Journal of Epidemiology* 90, no. 5 (1969): 406-415.

Meader, F.M., J.H. Means and J.G. Hopkins. "Account of an Epidemic of Influenza Among American Troops in England." *American Journal of the Medical Sciences* 158 (1919): 370-77.

Mears, Tim. "Acupuncture in the Treatment of Post Viral Fatigue Syndrome – a Case Report." *Acupuncture in Medicine* 23, no. 3 (September 2005): 141-45.

Ministry of Health, [London] United Kingdom. "The Influenza Epidemic in England and Wales, 1957-1958." *Reports on Public Health and Medical Subjects* 100 (1960).

Mishin, Vasily P., Frederick G. Hayden, Larisa V. Gubareva, "Susceptibilities of Antiviral-Resistant Influenza Viruses to Novel Neuraminidase Inhibitors," *Antimicrobial Agents and Chemotherapy* 49, no. 11 (November 2005): 4515-20.

Mote, John R., "Human and Swine Influenza," in *Virus and Rickettsial Diseases: With Especial Consideration of Their Public Health Significance.* Harvard School of Public Health Symposium, 12-17 June 1939. Cambridge: Harvard University Press, 1940.

Natelson, Benjamin H., Shelley A. Weaver, Chin-Lin Tseng, and John E. Ottenweller.

"Spinal Fluid Abnormalities in Patients with Chronic Fatigue Syndrome." *Clinical and Diagnostic Laboratory Immunology* 12, no. 1 (January 2005): 52-55.

Nicolle, Charles and C. Lebailly. *Comptes Rendus de l Academie des Sciences.* 1918, p. 607.

Opie, Eugene L. "The Pathologic Anatomy of Influenza: Based Chiefly on American and British Sources." *Archives of Pathology* 5 (1928): 285-303.

Opie, E. et al., "Pneumonia at Camp Funston." *Journal of the American Medical Association*, 72 (January 1919): 114-15.

Opie, Eugene Lindsay, Allen W. Freeman, Francis G. Blake, James C. Small, and Thomas M. Rivers. *Journal of the American Medical Association*, 11 January and 22 February 1919.

Osterholm, Michael T. "Preparing for the Next Pandemic." *New England Journal of Medicine* 352, no. 18, 5 May 2005, 1839-42.

Oxford, John S. "The So-called Great Spanish Influenza Pandemic of 1918 May Have Originated in France in 1916," *Philosophical Transactions of the Royal Society of London. Series B, Biological Sciences* 356, no. 1416, 29 December 2001, pp. 1857-59.

_____, Robert Lambkin, Armine Sefton, Rod Daniels, Aileen Elliot, R. Brown and D. Gill, "A Hypothesis: The Conjunction of Soldiers, Gas, Pigs, Ducks, Geese and Horses in Northern France During the Great War Provided the Conditions for the Emergence of the 'Spanish' Influenza Pandemic of 1918-1919," *Vaccine* 23, no. 7, 4 January 2005, pp. 940-45.

_____, Shobana Balasingham, Rob Lambkin, "A New Millennium Conundrum: How to Use a Powerful Class of Influenza Anti-Neuraminidase Drugs (NAIs) in the Community," *Journal of Antimicrobial Chemotherapy* 53 (2004): 133-36.

"Pneumonic Plague." (Editorial) *China Medical Journal* 32 (March 1918): 147-52.

"Pneumonic Plague in Nanking," *China Medical Journal* 32 (1918): 251-53.

Rachemann, Francis M. and Samuel Brock. "The Epidemic of Influenza at Camp Merritt, New Jersey." *Archives of Internal Medicine* 24 (1919): 582-602.

Red Cross Bulletin 2, 5 August 1918.

Regoes, Roland R. and Sebastian Bonhoeffer, "Emergence of Drug-Resistant Influenza Virus: Population Dynamical Considerations," *Science* 312, no. 5772, 21 April 2006, pp. 389-91.

"Report on Epidemic of Pneumonic Plague in Tsinanfu." *China Medical Journal* 32 (1918): 346-48.

Reid, Ann H. and Jeffery K. Taubenberger. "The Origin of the 1918 Pandemic Influenza Virus: A Continuing Enigma." *Journal of General Virology* 84, pt. 9 (September 2003): 2285-92.

"A Revised System of Nomenclature for Influenza Viruses." *Bulletin of the World Health Organization* 45 (1971): 119-24.

Rhodes, Lynwood Mark. "Killer on the Rampage: The Great Flu Epidemic." *Today's Health* 45 (October 1967): 24-27.

Rosenau, Milton Joseph. *Journal of the American Medical Association*, 2 August 1919.

Rosenow, E.C. "Studies in Influenza and Pneumonia." *Journal of Infectious Diseases* 26 (1920): 469-622.

Rybicka, Katarzyna and Lidia B. Brydak. "Encephalopathy and Encephalitis – Influenza -Associated Neurological Sequels." *Polski Merkuriusz Lekarski* 19 (October 2005): 501-05.

Schwarzmann, Stephen W., J.L. Adler, R.J. Sullivan, Jr., William M. Marine, "Bacterial Pneumonia During the Hong Kong Influenza Epidemic of 1968-1969," *Archives of Internal Medicine* 127, no. 6 (June 1971): 1037-41.

Shope, Richard E. "The Incidence of Neutralizing Antibodies for Swine Influenza Virus in the Sera of Human Beings of Different Ages." *Journal of Experimental Medicine* 63 (1936): 669-84.

Shreeve, Jamie. "Why Revive a Deadly Flu Virus?" *New York Times*, 29 January 2006.

Simonsen, Lone, Matthew J. Clarke, Lawrence B. Schonberger, Nancy H. Arden, Nancy J. Cox, and Keiji Fukuda. "Pandemic Versus Epidemic Influenza Mortality: A Pattern of Changing Age Distribution." *Journal of Infectious Diseases* 178 (1998): 53-60.

Smidt, M.H., H. Stroink, J.F. Bruinenberg, and M.F. Peeters. "Encephalopathy Associated with Influenza A." *European Journal of Paediatric Neurology* 8, no. 5 (2004): 257-60.

Smith, Wilson, C.H. Andrews, and Patrick Playfair Laidlaw. "A Virus Obtained from Influenza Patients." *Lancet* 225, 8 July 1933, 66-68.

Soper, George A. "The Pandemic in the Army Camps." *Journal of the American Medical Association* 71 (1918): 1899-1909.

_____. "Influenza in Horses and in Man." *New York Medical Journal* 109 (1919): 720-24.

"Sources of Influenza." *British Medical Journal* 2, 30 June 1973, 730-31.

Stanley, Arthur, M.D., [Health Officer, Shanghai Municipal Council, Public Health Report 1918], "Medical Reports," *China Medical Journal* 33 (1919): 273.

_____. "Notes on Pneumonic Plague in China." *China Medical Journal* 32 (May 1918): 207-09.

_____. "Medical Reports." *China Medical Journal* 33 (1919): 272-73.

Stephenson, Iain and Jane Democratis, "Influenza: Current Threat from Avian Influenza," *British Medical Bulletin* 75-76, no. 1 (2006): 63-80.

Stevens, James, Ola Blixt, L. Glaser, Jeffrey K. Taubenberger, Peter Palese, James C. Paulson, Ian A. Wilson, "Glycan Microarray Analysis of the Hemagglutinins from Modern and Pandemic Influenza Viruses Reveals Different Receptor Specificities," *Journal of Molecular Biology* 355 (February 2006): 1143-55.

_____, Ola Blixt, Terrence M. Tumpey, Jeffrey K. Taubenberger, James C. Paulson, Ian A. Wilson, "Structure and Receptor Specificity of the Haemagglutinin from an H5N1 Influenza Virus," *Science* 312, no. 5772, 21 April 2006, pp. 404-10.

Symmers, Douglas. "Pathologic Similarity Between Pneumonia of Bubonic Plague and of Pandemic Influenza." *Journal of the American Medical Association* 71, 2 November 1918, 1482-85.

Talon, Julie, Curt M. Horvath, Rosalind Polley, Christopher F. Basler, Thomas F. Muster, Peter Palese, and Adolfo Garcia-Sastre. "Activation of Interferon Regulatory Factor 3 is Inhibited by the Influenza A Virus NS1 Protein." *Journal of Virology* 74, no. 17 (September 2000): 7989-96.

Tashiro, Masato, Pawel S. Ciborowski, Hans Dieter Klenk, Gerhard Pulverer, and Rudolf Rott. "Role of Staphylococcus Protease in the Development of Influenza Pneumonia." *Nature* 325, 5 February 1987, 536-37.

Taubenberger, Jeffery K. "Chasing the Elusive 1918 Virus: Preparing for the Future by Examining the Past," in *The Threat of Pandemic Influenza, Are we Ready?: Workshop Summary*, eds. Stacey L. Knobler, Alison Mack, Adel Mahmoud, and Stanley M. Lemon. Washington, D.C.: National Academics Press, 2005.

Taubenberger, Jeffery K., Ann H. Reid and Thomas G. Fanning. "Capturing a Killer Flu Virus." *Scientific American* 292, no 1 (January 2005): 62-71.

Taubenberger, Jeffrey K., Ann H. Reid, Thomas A. Janczewski, and Thomas G. Fanning. "Integrating Historical, Clinical and Molecular Genetic Data in Order to Explain the Origin and Virulence of the 1918 Spanish Influenza Virus." *Philosophical Transactions of the Royal Society of London, Series B, Biological Sciences* 356, 29 December 2001, 1829-39.

Tognotti, Eugenia, "Scientific Triumphalism and Learning from Facts: Bacteriology and the "Spanish flu" Challenge of 1918," *Social History of Medicine* 16, no. 1 (2003): 97-110.

Torrea, Gabriela, Viviane Chenal-Francisque, Alexandre Leclercq, and Elisabeth Carniel. "Efficient Tracing of Global Isolates of *Yersinia pestis* by Restriction Fragment Length Polymorphism Analysis Using Three Insertion Sequences as Probes." *Journal of Clinical Microbiology* 44, no. 6 (June 2006): 2084-92.

Treanor, John J., James D. Campbell, Kenneth M. Zangwill, Thomas Rowe, M.S. Wolff and Mark Wolff, "Safety and Immunogenicity of an Inactivated Subvirion Influenza A (H5N1) Vaccine," *New England Journal of Medicine* 354, no. 13, p.9. (2006): 1347-51.

Tumpey, Terrence M., Christopher F. Basler, Patricia V. Aguilar, Hui Zeng, Alicia Solorzano, David E. Swayne, Nancy J. Cox, Jacqueline M. Katz, Jeffrey K. Taubenberger, Peter Palese, and Adolofo Garcia-Sastre. "Characterization of the Reconstructed 1918 Spanish Influenza Pandemic Virus." *Science* 310 no. 5745, 7 October 2005, 77-80.

"Twenty-Fifth Anniversary – Yale School of Nursing." *Yale Journal of Biology and Medicine* (1949): 264-71.

Uiprasertkul, Mongkol, Pilaipan Puthavathana, Kantima Sangsiriwut, Phisanu Pooruk, Kanittar Srisook, Malik Peiris, John M. Nicholls, Kulkanya Chokephaibulkit, Nirun Vanprapar, and Prasert Auewarakul. "Influenza A H5N1 Replication Sites in Humans." *Emerging Infectious Diseases* 11, no. 7 (July 2005): 1036-41.

Vaughan, Warren T. *Influenza: An Epidemiological Study*. Baltimore: *American Journal of Hygiene*, Monographic Series, No. 1, 1921.

Vu, David M., Alberdina W. de Boer, Lisa Danzig, George Santos, Bridget Canty, Betty M. Flores, and Dan M. Granoff. "Priming for Immunologic Memory in Adults by Meningococcal Group C Conjugate Vaccine." *Clinical and Vaccine Immunology* 13, no. 6 (June 2006): 605-10.

Webster, Robert G., "Predictions for Future Human Influenza Pandemics." *Journal of Infectious Diseases* 176, Suppl. 1 (August 1997): S14-19.

Weinstein, Edwin A. "Woodrow Wilson's Neurological Illness." *Journal of American History* 57 (1970-71): 324-51.

Westphal, Mary E. "Influenza Vignettes." *Public Health Nurse* 11, no. 2 (1919): 129-33.

Winslow, C.-E. A., and Rogers, J.F. "Statistics of the 1918 Epidemic of Influenza in Connecticut." *Journal of Infectious Diseases* 26 (1920): 185-216.

Writing Committee of the World Health Organization (WHO) Consultation on Human Influenza A/H5, "Avian Influenza A (H5N1) Infection in Humans," *New England Journal of Medicine* 353, no. 13, 29 September 2005, pp. 1374-85.

Young, Anne. "Clinical Similarity Between Influenza Epidemic and Plague." *New York Medical Journal* 109, 17 May 1919, 856-57.

Zinsser, Hans. "The Etiology and Epidemiology of Influenza." *Medicine* 1 (1922): 213-309.

UNPUBLISHED MATERIALS

Hattwick, Michael A.W., Chief, Respiratory and Special Pathogens Branch, Viral Diseases Division, Bureau of Epidemiology, Center for Disease Control. Interview by Dorothy Pettit, 24 March 1975, Atlanta, Georgia.

Hiscock, Ira Vaughan, Professor of Public Health, Emeritus, Yale University. Interview by Dorothy Pettit, 15 August 1975, New Haven, Connecticut.

Noyes, William Raymond. "Influenza Epidemic 1918-1919: A Misplaced Chapter in United States Social and Institutional History." Ph.D. dissertation, University of California, Los Angeles, 1968.

Serfling, Robert E., and Sherman, Ida L. "Excess Mortality During Influenza Epidemics in the United States, 1915-1962." Paper presented at the 1962 Annual Meeting of the American Public Health Association by the Chief Statistician of the Epidemiology Branch, Communicable Disease Center, Public Health Service, Atlanta, Georgia.

AUDIOVISUAL

Morrissey, Carla. *Influenza, 1918: The American Experience.* Directed by Matthew Collins. Arlington, Va.: A Robert Kenner Film Production, PBS Home Video, 14 April 1998.

GOVERNMENT PUBLICATIONS

U.S. Department of the Army. *The Medical Department of the United States Army in the World War,* by Maj. Gen. M.W. Ireland. Vol. 9. *Communicable and Other Diseases,* by Lieut. Col. Joseph F. Siler, M.C., U.S. Army. Washington, D.C.: Government Printing Office, 1928.

U.S. Department of the Army. Historical Division. *United States Army in the World War 1917-1919.* Reports of the Commander-in-Chief, A.E.F., Staff Sections and Services. Washington, D.C.: Government Printing Office, 1948.

U.S. Department of Commerce. Bureau of the Census. *Special Tables of Mortality from Influenza and Pneumonia in Indiana, Kansas, and Philadelphia, Pa. September 1 to December 31, 1918.* Washington, D.C.: Government Printing Office, 1920.

U.S. Department of Health, Education, and Welfare. Public Health Service. *Mortality from Influenza and Pneumonia in 50 Large Cities of the United States 1910-1929,* by Selwyn D. Collins, W.H. Frost, Mary Gover, and Edgar Sydenstricker. Reprint No. 1415 from *Public Health Reports.* Washington, D.C.: Government Printing Office.

U.S. Department of Health, Education, and Welfare. Public Health Service. *Excess Deaths from Influenza and Pneumonia and from Important Chronic Diseases During Epidemic Periods 1918-1951,* by Selwyn D. Collins and Josephine Lehman. Public Health Service Publication No. 213. Washington, D.C.: Government Printing Office, 1953.

U.S. Department of Health, Education, and Welfare. Public Health Service. "Trend and Age Variation of Mortality and Morbidity from Influenza and Pneumonia," in *Long-Time Trends in Illness and Medical Care.* Public Health Monograph No. 48, 1957.

U.S. Department of Health, Education, and Welfare. National Institutes of Health, Bethesda, Maryland. *The Study of Influenza,* by B.V. Zhdanov, V.D. Solon'ev, and F.G. Epshtein. A translation of *Ucheniye o Grippe* by L.L. Fadeyeva, 1958. Prepared and distributed by the Russian Scientific Translation Program, Division of General Medical Sciences, National Institutes of Health, 1960.

U.S. Department of Labor. *Annual Report of the Commissioner General of Immigration to the Secretary of Labor.* Fiscal Years ended June 30, 1918 to June 30, 1922. Washington, D.C.: Government Printing Office, 1922.

U.S. Department of Labor. Bureau of Labor Statistics. *Chinese Migrations, with Special Reference to Labor Conditions*, by Ta Chen. Bulletin of the U.S. Bureau of Labor Statistics No. 340. Washington, D.C.: Government Printing Office, 1923.

U.S. Department of the Navy. Bureau of Medicine and Surgery. *Annual Report of the Surgeon General, U.S. Navy (1919)*. Washington, D.C.: Government Printing Office, 1919.

NEWSPAPERS

Billboard, 1918-20.

China Weekly Review (Shanghai), 1917-18.

Louisville (Kentucky) *Courier Journal*, 1919.

New Haven (Conn.) *Journal Courier*, 1977-78.

New York American, 1918.

New York Telegram, 1919.

New York Times, 1917-20.

North China Herald and Supreme Court and Consular Gazette (Shanghai), 1917-18.

Washington, D.C., *Evening Star, 1919*

Washington Post, 1917-20.

Yale Daily News, 1918-20.

Index

F

G

Gravedigger shortage, 110–111
Grayson, Cary T., 164, 169, 171–172, 216
S.S. *Great Northern*, 156
Grenfell, Bryan T., 249
Grew, Joseph, 158, 159, 160
Grief, from illness and war, 174–175, 226–228
Grippe. *see* Influenza
Gross, Henry, 168
Guillain-Barré syndrome, 245

H

Haddad, Michael, 116
Haddad, Paul, 116
Haddad, Peter, 116
Hadley, Arthur T., 192
Haemophilus influenzae, 26, 27
Hard colds. *see* Influenza
Harding, Warren G., 223, 225–226, 249
Harriman, Daisy, 161, 162
Harriman, J. Borden, 136
Harvard unit, 69
Haskell County, Kansas, 232
Hawkes, Herbert E., 191
Health care
    in Cincinnati, 181, 182, 183
    education, 189–192
    hospital facilities. *see* Hospitals and care facilities
    nursing training, 186–189
    public health. *see* Public health
    quality of care. *see* Quality of care
    rehabilitation hospitals, 194
Heart conditions, 181, 191
Hemagglutinin (HA), 6–7, 8, 14, 34, 235, 240
Hemingway, Dr. [Clarence Edmonds], 90
Hiccoughs, 226
Hinckley, Thomas, 154
Hines, Walker D., 214

Hiscock, Ira V., 68, 69f
Hog flu. *see* Swine flu
Holmes, Edward C., 249
Holt, Emmet, 190
Hong Kong influenza, 12, 17t
Hoover, Herbert, 164
Hoover, Ike, 169
Hope, in 1920, 205, 226
Hospitals and care facilities
    on Armistice day, 136
    at Camp Devens, 86–87
    at Camp Pike, 142
    emergency hospitals, 45f, 49f, 82f, 108, 144
    in France, run by Joseph Aub, 37
    German, 72, 73, 74
    Hopkins' Base Hospital No. 18, 81–82
    hygiene and preventive measures, 45
    investigation and inadequacy of, 39–42, 90, 95, 106
    Johns Hopkins, 119
    nursing availability, 186
    preparedness, 247
    rehabilitation and rest hospitals, 194
    shortage of space, 88–90, 92–95, 106
    treatment of post-influenzal conditions, 174
    U.S. Army Influenza Hospital officers, 56f
    on U.S.S. *Khiva*, 68
    Washington D.C. area hospitals, 106, 108, 144
House, Edward M.
    on Armistice signing, 135, 159
    on death of Gunner Flodin, 160
    on death of Willard Straight, 162
    illness of, 46
    peace term negotiations on behalf of President, 172
    photograph of, 121f
    recovery in health, 161–162

309